YOUR
BIG FAT
BOYFRIEND

Library of Congress Cataloging in Publication Number:
2008929115

ISBN: 978-1-59474-290-3

Printed in China

Typeset in Helvetica

Designed by Bryn Ashburn
Illustrations by Neryl Walker
Edited by Sarah O'Brien

Distributed in North America by Chronicle Books
680 Second Street
San Francisco, CA   94107

10 9 8 7 6 5 4 3 2 1

Quirk Books
215 Church Street
Philadelphia, PA 19106
www.quirkbooks.com

YOUR BIG FAT BOYFRIEND

How to Stay Thin When Dating a Diet Disaster

by Jenna Bergen

QUIRK BOOKS
PHILADELPHIA

TABLE OF
CONTENTS

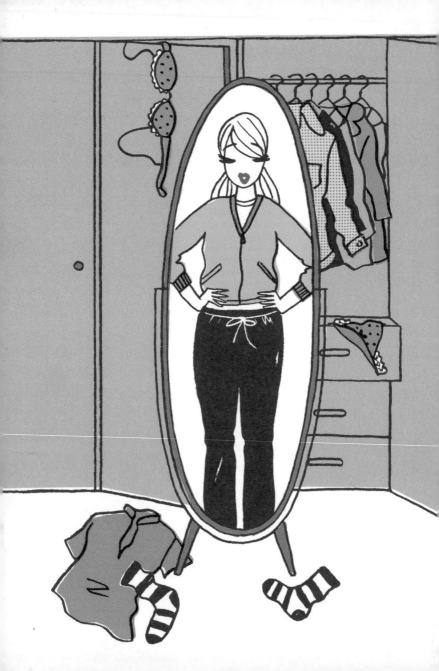

CHAPTER 1

THE DOWNWARD
SLIDE INTO FAT PANTS

I still remember "the moment." That awful, clarifying instant when I realized I'd gone from thin to not-so-thin. It was a freezing Friday in February, and it had been, quite completely, the day from hell. I'd intended to leave the office early and arrive home in time to wash and blow-dry my hair, shave my legs, and look verifiably amazing by the time he rang the bell at 8 P.M.

I walk in the door at 7:45 with coffee on my shirt and a run in my stockings nearing hooker proportions. I'm on a mission to look good and look good fast: My boyfriend—we'll leave names out of this story in order to protect the incriminated—is on his way to pick me up for a little après workweek dinner. Which is why, at 7:50, I am on my knees, halfway into my closet, blindly searching for my totally hot, erase-ten-pounds, make-my-ass-look-amazing jeans. Where are they? I need to feel hot, attractive, desirable—instantly. I need those jeans.

While unearthing the bottom of my closet, I spot one jean leg dangling over the back of my desk chair. I lunge toward the chair, feeling a shot of relief course though my body as I confirm: We have liftoff. They are the jeans.

They're a little wrinkly, but they'll work. I shake them violently—my only form of ironing—and then shove in my right foot and try to yank on the leg as I hop toward the closet to grab my go-to black V-neck.

Ooh, that's weird, I think, as I struggle to pull the denim up and over my thighs. Suddenly, a terrible feeling washes over me. *They feel too tight.*

I wedge my hands into the front pockets and push the denim away from my body. I do a deep squat, attempting to loosen the material. There's no give—they don't fit. I try to channel my yoga instructor and breathe deeply. *Don't panic. Just take a breath . . .*

No. They *have* to fit. I violently pull the V-neck over my head and yank down the hem, trying to cover the now-lumpy bulge that should have been my waist.

I look at my reflection in the mirror. I try to reason with myself. *I have them on. The button still fits through the hole, so, technically, they fit.* But just barely. I turn to the side and check out my profile. Instead of being perfectly snug around all the right curves, they're tight *everywhere*, and I have an unattractive, extra bit of myself hanging over the top of my jeans.

I suck in, hollowing out my stomach and puffing out my chest. The result is no better: I look like some sort of disproportionate linebacker. I exhale loudly and my spine sinks back to its normal five foot four frame and the excess belly reappears. My thighs look painted in denim. This cannot be happening.

My mind frantically tries to problem solve: *Maybe I can get away with wearing them. With a loose, flowy top and some cute heels, maybe no one will notice.* I stiffly walk to my bed. I attempt to sit. *Ow. Okay, no.* There's no way these are going to work. Not unless I want to sit like a statue hoping the crotch doesn't rip while I sip on nothing but lemon water all night.

I am hopping on one foot again, but this time in a frantic attempt to peel off the right pant leg. I lose my balance and fall sideways onto the bed, where I continue my totally unattractive struggle to remove the spiteful clothing from my body. *Finally!* I toss the offending jeans across the room and flop onto my back, staring up at the ceiling wearing only my bra, underwear, and a frown.

How had this happened? How had I gone from wearing

cute, adorable jeans and tight tanks every night to *this*?
I work out. I am the *queen* of veggies.

Maybe it was the dryer, my kind, compassionate little
ego tries to console me.

No. It wasn't the dryer. I remember a time three
months ago when I'd pulled on the very same jeans. They
had been snug, but wearable. Still, that night I had opted
for total comfort and grabbed my super-soft sweatpants
instead. Why be anything but totally relaxed? My honey
and I were just going to spend the evening watching
movies and eating takeout. . .

My mind flashes to nights of us sitting side by side
on the couch as I happily neglect my chicken and string
beans and share his sesame chicken straight from the
box; forgoing my light beer for a full-bodied brew he
wants me to try; sharing not just popcorn, but popcorn,
candy, *and* soda at the movies; matching him bite for
bite on the calamari or baskets of nacho chips he talked
me into ordering; allowing him to pull me back under the
covers instead of making it to my yoga class. *Oh my
God—it's him!*

"I never used to order appetizers!" I yell, with only
my walls to hear me. I hop off the bed and scurry to the
bathroom. I hate scales and I hate weighing myself; and
I have a strong belief it's not really necessary if you're
working out and eating healthfully, but I knew the time

had come. I braced myself. I closed my eyes. I took a breath, tried to make myself as light as humanly possible, reminded myself it had been three hours since I had last peed, and then looked down.

My naked feet bracketed the red numbers on the scale. Holy Lord, Hail Mary — 13 pounds!

It was then, at that moment, that I realized something: I didn't just have a BF. I had an FB! No, not even. A *B*FB. I was dating a Big. Fat. Boyfriend.

I ADMIT, I HAD WARNING SIGNS

We were in the same class at college. I always came directly from the gym, wearing my Ithaca sweatshirt, hair pulled back in a messy ponytail, sipping water to rehydrate after my 45-minute elliptical jaunt. Each morning he rolled into class with earphones filling his ears and a sleepy, just-rolled-out-of-bed kind of cool. He was adorable, with big brown eyes, a mop of thick, just-curly-enough-that-you-want-to-touch-it hair, and he hardly spoke a word. Half of me wanted to ask him about his writing, but the other half was put off (okay, repulsed) by his mid-morning eating habits. While I plopped down my notebooks and apple, he procured a Snickers and a caramel Twix. He'd unwrap one, down it in four bites, and be on to number two before our professor even had her papers situated. And each morning, I watched him with a sort of disgusted fascination.

"That's your breakfast?" I finally asked him one day, as other students were still filing in.

"Yep." His eyes met mine for the first time. He smiled. I wrinkled my nose in feminine disgust. Still, we hit it off, and the images of discarded candy bar wrappers soon faded from my memory.

However, I knew something was definitely wrong with him on our first date, when he efficiently fished out all the bits of celery and carrot from his cup of chicken noodle. "I hate vegetables," he told me, when he noticed me eyeing the growing pile on his saucer. And then he grinned, a smile so adorable that at that moment I could not have cared less if he ate vats of lard for every meal.

His total abhorrence for anything healthy might have been okay, had I been stronger—as in, inhuman. I started out armed with my health-conscious ways, but the longer we were together, the happier I was with him, and the easier it was to slip into the cohabitating habits of nibbling from his plate, polishing off the bread basket, and snacking on whatever goodies were in his cupboards.

Even more dangerously, the more I knew we loved each other, the less I cared that he held onto the false assumption that there was anything truly dainty about me. So I said goodbye to eating only a few bites of dinner or to feigning fullness when he offered a late-night snack. No, I hadn't give up all of my yummy veggies and big green salads I honestly enjoyed, but I had started adding a lot of tastes here and nibbles there of his high-fat, always-fried, not-a-low-carb-item-in-the-bunch foods. And those little allowances had added up to 13 big ones.

THANKFULLY, I WASN'T ALONE

The influence of partners on eating behaviors has been studied around the world—from the United States and the United Kingdom to Finland and Australia. When I started sharing my weighty news with other women, I found that lots of girls were gaining much more than a new best friend when meeting their BF.

"Jon is the greatest guy you could ever date," says Lindsey, 20. "He is sweet, attentive, and devoted. But his diet—and mine—is as inconsistent and on-and-off as Pam and Tommy Lee!" The two started dating in high school, when working out and eating right was the last thing on their minds, and they bonded over everything from nachos to Pop-Tarts. But after four years and a 20-pound jump on the scale, Lindsey realized it had gone too far. "Everything clung to me in all the wrong places," she recalls. "I wanted to crawl out of my own skin."

Food habits are influenced by many factors throughout your life, including your parents, where you're brought up, your socioeconomic status, and who you date. "Having a boyfriend or moving in together is a big, significant, life-changing event," says Amelia Lake, a registered dietician and post-doctoral fellow at the Human Nutrition Research Centre at Newcastle University, England. "It has quite an impact on your life."

Multiple studies have been done about this couple-cushioning factor. Although most have focused on married and cohabitating couples, dating can have the same effect, because it brings together two individuals who have different habits, hunger cues, and food choices. "Food and eating are really important parts of our culture, especially as a couple," says Lake. "You eat out together, you go to the cinema together. And we live in a society where you can go to a Starbucks and buy a drink that is half your daily energy requirements."

Food begins to have more meaning, too. With hectic schedules—whether it's long hours at the office or other tugs and pulls from family and friends—many couples use dinner as a way to spend more time with one another. "Meals become more symbolic," says Lake. "There's an importance placed on eating together." Which, she says, can lead couples to eat more than they would if they were eating alone.

Perhaps the most frustrating factor is that while you pack on the pounds, your man has a good chance of *losing* weight. Research shows that living with a male puts pressure on females to consume more unhealthy foods, whereas females have a positive influence on the diets of their partners. "I think it's about practicality," says Lake. "If you love chocolate but wouldn't necessarily buy it, but he buys it so it's now freely available, chances are, you're going to eat it." So, while you strive to eat healthy and keep him from meeting an early death by stocking the fridge with fruits and veggies, you can't help but succumb to his burgers and fries. This imbalance can wreak havoc on your waistline—and set you up for health problems later. "It's not just about being paranoid if your bum looks big," says Lake. "This can affect your long-term health."

SO, WHAT'S A GIRL TO DO?

As I sat there that night waiting for my BFB to escort me to dinner—with seam imprints running the length of my thighs—I realized that no matter how awful his eating habits were, I couldn't give up on our relationship just to avoid love handles. But the time had come to pull out every stay-slim trick in the book—I wasn't about to let go of my pre-BFB body so easily.

I grabbed a little black dress (wonderfully unrestrictive and still sweetly sexy), pulled my hair back, swiped on mascara, dabbed on some lip gloss—and hoped to God I could keep my hands off his fries at dinner.

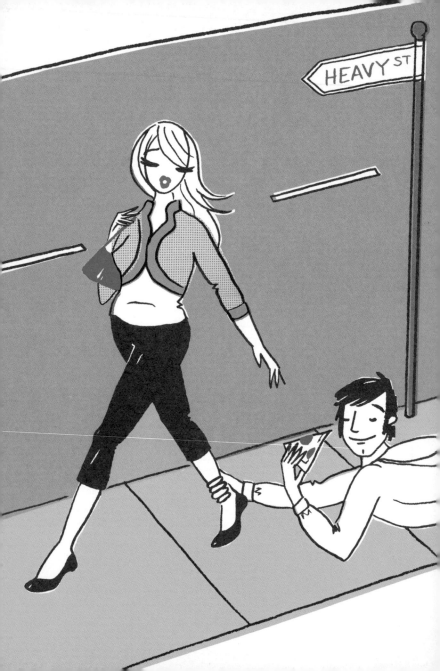

CHAPTER 2

WHY HE'S
WEIGHING YOU DOWN

I see him trying to get my attention while I peruse the protein bars. One aisle over, he's holding up some sort of fruit pie and waving it at me. We're standing in a convenience store, it's not even a quarter past 8 A.M., and he's proposing a sugar- and fat-laden dessert for breakfast.

"Those have about 500 calories," I tell him.

He flips the package over and, for a second, I feel proud that he now knows that nutritional information does, in fact, exist.

"Four-hundred eighty! That's amazing. How did you know that?"

I shrug, proud of myself for retaining this bit of info. "You know sports stats and every Pink Floyd album in chronological order. *I* know nutritional facts." I expect him to put the package back on the rack. He doesn't.

"Well, 480's not that bad," he tells me. "You're supposed to have 20,000 calories a day."

Time freezes. The Slurpee machine stops churning and a woman's change suspends in midair. I stare at the love of my life in shock. Twenty—did I hear him right? Did he just say *20,000 calories a day*? My mind is reeling, struggling to comprehend how this intelligent, witty, and otherwise capable man can be this calorically challenged.

This is not, by any stretch, the first time we've talked about basic health and nutrition. We're *three* years into our relationship. I am a health *freak*. How does he not know the most fundamental of facts?! A helpful—and, obviously, totally overlooked—message that's been stamped on every box of cereal he's ever emptied: "Percent Daily Values are based on a 2,000 calorie diet." Has he been walking through life believing 1,000 calories is snack-size?

My last thought is so horrifying that I'm suddenly sucked back to the overly bright convenience store. I no longer care that the man behind the counter is watching with reality-TV-like interest.

"Twenty thousand? Try *two thousand*." My voice is so

cold it could strike fear into the hearts of unhealthy eaters everywhere. A man at the pastry case backs away from the doughnuts. He grabs a banana instead.

My darling, however, is not fazed. "Two thousand? That's nothing. I bet I could eat that in one meal." I shake my head, totally sure he could—and sadly, that I would put away at least half of whatever he was having, too.

"It's breakfast. It's supposed to be good for you," I say, parroting moms everywhere in one final, last-ditch attempt. Surprisingly, he concedes, putting the pie back on the shelf. I relax for a moment, the first diet disaster of the morning averted. Ha. This is no amateur I'm dealing with. I turn around with our coffees to find him holding a huge, could-feed-a-mini-van-of-eight coffee cake.

"Look, this one is only 390." He smiles, plopping the weighty cake on the counter beside our coffees. "I just saved 90 calories. It's like I spent 25 minutes on the treadmill." The cashier rings up our food as I shake my head, defeated. My BFB playfully elbows me in the side. I elbow him back, trying my best to sound stern.

"You're impossible."

His smile breaks down the big, huge, food-pyramid wall between us. "I'll still let you have a bite."

Yes, I know. That's exactly what I was afraid of.

THE TOP TEN REASONS YOUR BOYFRIEND IS ADDING BAGGAGE TO YOUR BACKSIDE

1 **He's a guy.** His mind stores sports stats and music trivia like a sponge sucks up water—not health and nutrition facts. No matter how often you tell him, prod him, or throw up your hands and scream, his mind will not hold onto the following words: fat, calories, daily allowances, nutrients, vitamins, antioxidants, or food groups. "He eats like a lineman," says Ciara, 20, who felt ill watching her ex-BFB down artery-clogging food each time they went out. "Cheesesteaks, that's it." She shudders, recalling how she would eat the cheese-filled submarines right along with him.

2 **He can *always* eat.** He just consumed a humongous lunch. An hour later, he's hungry. Again. And while his metabolism burns faster than a head full of hairspray, allowing him to shovel in huge quantities of food without affecting his bod, *you* have to spend 30 minutes on the treadmill to burn off a single piece of chocolate. "Dave could probably eat a horse," says Emily, 26. "And, much to my dismay, he would still fit into his little 32-inch-waist pants!" Her hollow-legged boyfriend has done everything from stop for fried chicken after downing an enormous lunch to almost shutting down a buffet. "Roast beef, fried chicken, ham, shrimp, salad, soup, a brownie sundae, peanut-butter pie. I don't think there was anything at that place he *didn't* eat."

(3) **Big is better.** His palms are almost three times the size of your little hands, and his idea of a "serving" is equally as large. "I eat more when I'm with him because he orders a larger meal," says Elena, 21, who credits her five-pound gain to weekend dinners with her BFB. "If I'm at a restaurant with a girlfriend, we usually finish eating around the same time because we both have similar meals. But when I'm with him, I continue to eat even though I'm no longer hungry because I'm waiting for him to finish."

(4) **You're his new BFF.** You love him, he loves you, and you've secured a spot in his top five. You're now the first person he thinks to call—about everything. The new job, an argument he had with a coworker, what gift to get his mom, and even for those really, really important things like who's kicking ass in fantasy hockey. Sure, it's fun. But this new title of BFF is heavy—pun intended—with responsibility. You're also his first call for midnight fast-food runs or grabbing wings and pints for Sunday night football.

"He used to love getting McDonald's for dinner," says Lisa, 21, who gained about 10 pounds due to a past BFB's fast-food addiction. "He'd even pick me up late at night from my sorority house to go get some. And it's way too hard to resist the smell of McDonald's! I would always order something, whether it was just fries or chicken nuggets, fries, *and* an apple pie!" Even after they broke up, it took Lisa months to kick the fast-food habit. "I would sometimes go on my own," she recalls. "I had never eaten fast food that much in my life."

5 **He thinks dieting is dumb.** A girl who pounds beers with the boys or is as excited as he is over the three-pizzas-for-$10 deal is much cooler than a dieting diva who refuses to eat anything other than rice cakes. "I didn't want to be that annoying girlfriend who picked at a salad instead of hunkering into a burger," says Emily, 25, who often found herself at a late-night diner with her BFB and his friends, surrounded by fries, mozzarella sticks, buffalo wings, and every other greasy-spoon favorite. "I wanted to be the cool, laid-back girlfriend who could be one of the guys," she remembers. "So while other dates were nibbling on salads and drinking seltzer, I was eating a burger and drinking a beer." Of course, those late nights started to show up in places other than her tired eyes.

6 **He loves you in sweatpants.** Nothing is better than finding a guy who loves you just as much in heels and a skimpy top as he does when you're lounging in front of the TV in baggy sweats and a T-shirt. Of course, lounging usually comes with snacking. "I live with my boyfriend, so a lot of our time is spent at home," says Erin, 25, who knows that no longer feeling the need to impress her BFB has caused her to put on weight. "I go from work clothes to sweats and sweat-shirts—it's hard to be comfy and snuggly in your skinny jeans and Jimmy Choos!" Of course, with that extra room comes room to grow, says Erin, recalling Saturday nights when she finally pulled out her dressy clothes only to find they were too tight. "In the worst-case scenario, you make it through Saturday night holding in your gut and standing up very straight," she laughs. "And then on Sunday, the sweats come out again and it starts all over."

7 **He's too cozy with the couch.** Don't be sur-prised if the last time he swung a racket was playing Wii. If you've got your own personal lazy boy, it's safe to assume the most weekend movement he'll muster is the short path between the couch and the fridge— and the chances of burning any calories with him are slim. "When I had a boyfriend, most of my spare time was spent with him instead of at the gym," says Lauren, 22, whose past BFB enjoyed watching sports or going out drinking. "Since we broke up, I lost about six pounds because I started eating healthier and working out more."

8 **Cooking = takeout.** Unless you're one of the lucky few who dates a chef, the extent of your boyfriend's culinary skills is grilled cheese, Ramen noodles, and a drawer stuffed full of takeout menus. "My boyfriend's apartment shared a street corner with every fast-food joint you can name: McDonald's, Taco Bell, Sonic, Pizza Hut, KFC," says Stephanie, 24. "He thought it was heaven; I thought it was the sixth circle of hell! I feared for my thighs!" After each visit, Stephanie hit the gym to work off the terrible takeout.

9 **He shops like a five-year-old.** Now that Mom's not around to keep the fridge filled, there's a good chance he's living out his childhood fantasy and buying every snack food he pleases. One hundred-calorie packs? Please. One foot inside his place and you're held captive by bottomless bags of mania-inducing munchies. "Pop-Tarts and Lucky Charms: there is never anything to eat in his apartment except those two items," says Carly, 21. "And maybe some chips or cookies. It makes it extremely hard to eat healthy."

10 The only "veggie" he eats is fried. If broccoli is his kryptonite, chances are that his plate will be filled with foods you'd normally avoid. "His love of cheese, bacon, and everything fried means that there are no vegetables allowed—unless they're covered in lard," says Chelsea, 23, who knows she eats way healthier when her BFB is not around. "He's a six-foot-five, 235-pound, former Division I lacrosse player—he eats Chalupas and KFC bowls in multiples of three!"

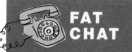

FAT CHAT

COMPLAINTS ABOUT BAD HABITS FROM REAL WOMEN LIKE YOU

Besides the flowers and love notes, these women have received something else from their wonderful BFBs. Here are just a few of the horrible habits they've picked up now that they're sharing saliva.

"Drinking milkshakes before bed!" —Emily, 25

"Thinking that I can lose weight as quickly as he does." —Carly, 21

"Cheetos." —Carrie, 30

"NOT dieting or exercising. Hah." —Samantha, 22

"Eating late at night." —Lauren, 22

"Fast food and drinking juice instead of water." —Jill, 28

"Choosing fried food when we're out." —Melissa, 26

"Red meat!" —Mandy, 28

"To be a yo-yo dieter." —Lindsey, 20

"A sweet tooth." —Becky, 19

"Drinking alcohol and high-calorie food." —Christina, 22

"Eat more, exercise less." —Sue, 21

"Putting half a jar of mayo on a BLT." —Jessica, 23

SPOT YOUR MAN

Who you're dealing with: The fast-food fan

How to spot him: The McDonald's cup in the car or the burger wrappers overflowing from the trashcan.

Why he's trouble: Fast food meals pack loads of calories and are crazy high in salt and saturated fat.

How to deal: Check out the calorie content of his favorite places online and find a few less destructive options for nights you can't avoid the drive-thru. If it's a new spot, opt for unsweetened iced tea and grilled chicken, and say no to fries.

• •

Who you're dealing with: An anti-veggie

How to spot him: He spot-checks his food before chowing down to make sure none of the good-for-him offenders have snuck their way onto his plate.

Why he's trouble: If he's avoiding greens, his plate will undoubtedly be filled with high-carb and high-fat foods like pasta, chicken fingers, and fries.

How to deal: Make sure to fill up on lots of veggies when you're not with him, so on nights when he cooks you meat and well, more meat, you'll have already met your daily quota.

• •

Who you're dealing with: The hollow leg

How to spot him: He's almost always chewing something and has snacks stashed everywhere around his house.

Why he's trouble: Just seeing food can make a girl hungry. So the more he's eating, the more inclined you are to nosh with him.

How to deal: Gum is a girl's best friend. If you've already eaten, pop a piece to avoid reflexive nibbling.

Who you're dealing with: The inhaler

How to spot him: By the time you turn around with the drinks, his plate is clean. Sometimes he is spotted with food on his shirt or chin.

Why he's trouble: You feel compelled to keep up with him and don't have time to register when you're really full.

How to deal: Realize that you're eating faster than normal, slow down, and encourage him to keep you company while you finish.

....

Who you're dealing with: The junk-food junkie

How to spot him: Open his cupboards. If you find that candy bars, potato chips, and ice cream are his staples, he's probably an addict.

Why he's trouble: If it's there, you're going to want to eat it.

How to deal: Eat before you stop by his place so you're not starving when you get there.

....

Who you're dealing with: The food pusher

How to spot him: He constantly insists that you try his burger, his milkshake, or other fatty foods you'd never let past your lips otherwise.

Why he's trouble: You feel compelled to try it, even if you're not hungry.

How to deal: After you decline his first offer, let him know that you'll ask him for a bite if you change your mind. And if it's really something you don't want to eat, claim allergies.

BFB FINAL THOUGHT

His "you're perfect just the way you are" bit might not be helpful for staying slim . . . but it sure is nice to hear sometimes.

I've been trying on different outfits for almost 20 minutes now, but I can't help it. I feel . . . fat. I sigh, loudly.

My BFB looks up from his laptop. "I liked the first one you had on."

"I feel like I've gained 10 pounds!" I dramatically flop onto the bed. "Hand me your sweatshirt. I'll wear big, voluminous clothes for the rest of my life."

"Stop, you'll be the hottest girl there. Five pounds, ten pounds . . . I can't tell that stuff."

I sigh, relenting a bit. He can tell he's broken through and tosses me a shirt. I guess he's right. I do look fine. He smacks my ass on the way to the door. "Come on, hottie, let's go. I'm hungry."

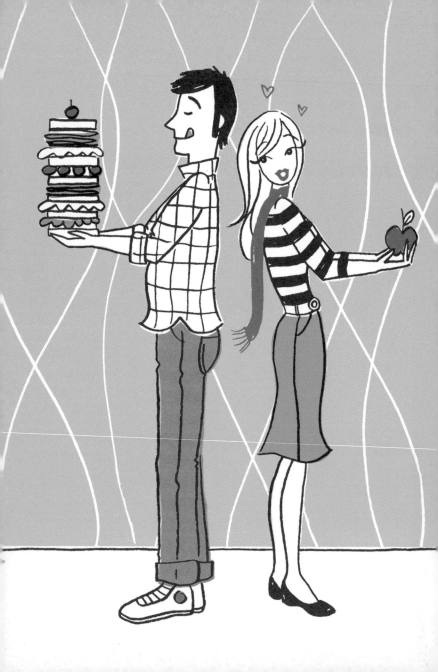

CHAPTER 3

THE HARD TRUTH:
YOU CAN'T EAT LIKE A MAN
(AND STILL FIT IN YOUR PANTS)

We plop down into our seats at a Mets–Phillies game. My BFB is checking out the starting pitchers in the bullpen, but all I can think about is how much I need a drink. It's beyond hot tonight.

"This is gonna be a great game." My BFB leans back in the seat and notices I look less than enthusiastic. "Thirsty?" he asks.

He waves down a vendor who hands over two ice-cold light beers. The vendor eyes us up: me in my Phillies cap and my BFB in his Mets gear. We're as night and day as they come.

The first crack of the bat sounds and it's suddenly three innings in. Beer has never tasted so good. I'm on my second bottle and my BFB has just returned holding a carrier overflowing with hot dogs, nachos, peanuts, and I don't even want to know what else. He hands me a dog.

I take it, wondering when I last ate such a processed, fat-filled frank. He sees me inspecting it.

"C'mon, it's a ball game. You gotta eat this stuff; it's half the fun." He angles the nachos toward me. I take one and dip into the totally fake cheese. Not bad, I have to admit. Tastes pretty damn good with the beer, the dog, and the baseball surroundings.

The innings move with the lazy pace of summer, and I start to slow on my ball game–induced chow down. My BFB, however, is still going strong. He offers me a peanut.

"No, thanks. Aren't you getting full?" I ask.

"I'm still getting a cheesesteak."

I shake my head in disbelief and wonder how he doesn't weigh 400 pounds. "Don't you ever worry about heart disease? Hypertension?" He jumps up to cheer as some Reyes guy makes a double play. I remember I'm talking to a guy wearing *Mets* gear to a *Phillies* game and realize death doesn't factor in much to his thought process.

He waves down the vendor for another round, and I envision us up on the JumboTron as they announce the couple that's consumed the most calories by the seventh-inning stretch. The crowd cheers, the Phillie Phanatic taunts us with a "look how fat they are" dance, and my BFB lets out a whoop, pumping his hand in the air and lifting his shirt, proudly showing off his belly to the packed stands. I sink down in my chair and try to hide behind the oversized box of popcorn. Which might have worked had I not consumed enough salt to puff me up to the size of the Goodyear blimp.

"He was outta lights," my BFB informs me as he hands me a regular beer. I take it and tell him that after this one, I'm tapping out. He shakes his head as if I've somehow let him down and I realize that I will never be able to consume as many calories as this kid—a fact that my ass is incredibly thankful for. But, at the same time, what I just ate was still way too much for my body.

I had to face facts. I'm a girl, and he's a guy. Although I will fight him to the death to win any game, I am *way* better at planning ahead, and I can kill a bug without crying (I never said he was brave), he has me beat when it comes to how much food we put away.

Let's face it: Unless you want to have his beefy bod, you need to eat a little less beef than he does. It all comes down to basic chemistry.

THE BASIC FACTS

You can thank one word for the reason you should never match your man bite for bite: *testosterone*. The hormone that makes your man a man is the main reason behind his (annoying) ability to eat so much without gaining a single ounce. That's because this hyperactive hormone causes the body to build lean muscle mass, and a pound of muscle burns more calories at rest (read: while he's on the couch) than a pound of fat.

"It's just biology," says Kathleen Zelman, a registered dietician and director of nutrition for WebMD Health and the WebMD Weight Loss Clinic. She explains that guys are genetically wired to be able to consume more food than women; "Calorie levels are primarily based on muscle mass, and guys were designed with a higher percentage." Women, on the other hand, were designed—genetically speaking—for pregnancy, and therefore they carry more body fat. So think of your BFB as a gas-sucking SUV and yourself as an energy-saving hybrid. They are bigger, they weigh more, and they require more energy to sustain their hulking muscle mass.

The number of calories you need daily depends on your age, your activity level, and how much lean muscle mass you're toting. On average, Zelman says girls need between 1,600 and 2,400 calories per day and guys need 2,000 to 3,000. Even if you and your man were the same age, height, and weight, he would still be able to put away 200–300 calories more than you each day, just because he's got bigger muscles. It's not the least bit fair, but it's true.

For a more specific idea of how many calories you can eat each day to maintain your current weight, grab a calculator. Use the following formula to find your basal metabolic rate (BMR)— how many calories your body burns every 24 hours to simply keep you alive and breathing. If you have a lot of muscle or very little muscle, the equation may under- or overestimate your caloric needs.

WOMEN'S BMR

655 + (4.35 x weight in pounds) + (4.7 x height in inches) – (4.7 x age in years) For example, a woman who weighs 135 pounds, is 5′4″, and is 25 years old has a equation that looks like this:

655 + (4.35 x 135) + (4.7 x 64) – (4.7 x 25)

①Do the math inside the parentheses first:

4.35 x 135 = 587.25, 4.7 x 64 = 300.8, 4.7 x 25 = 117.5

②Then plug the numbers back into the equation:

655 + 587.25 + 300.8 – 117.5 = 1425.55

So this woman needs 1,425.55 calories each day to

maintain her current weight if she does nothing but sit on the couch for 24 hours.

To factor in daily exercise, multiply your BMR by one of the following:

- **Sedentary (little or no exercise):** BMR x 1.2
- **Lightly active (light exercise 1–3 days per week):** BMR x 1.375
- **Moderately active (moderate exercise 3–5 days per week):** BMR x 1.55
- **Very active (hard exercise 6–7 days a week):** BMR x 1.725
- **Extra active (very hard exercise and a physical job):** BMR x 1.9

If our 25-year-old example is moderately active, we multiply her BMR by 1.55: 1425.55 x 1.55 = 2,209.6

So she can consume about 2,200 calories a day without gaining weight. Now she can figure out how many calories to cut each day to lose weight. If she trims her calories back to 1,800 a day, she'll save 400 calories a day. And if 1 pound equals 3,500 calories, she'll lose a pound about every nine days. Just remember, as you lose weight, you'll need to rework these formulas to find out what your new caloric requirements are, since they'll go down as you lose weight.

BFBs can find their BMR with this equation, specifically formulated for men:

MEN'S BMR

66 + (6.23 x weight in pounds) + (12.7 x height in inches) – (6.8 x age in years)

They can use the same formula to factor in their activity levels.

EASY GAINS

If it seems like you've been putting on weight since meeting Mr. Right, there's a very good reason. Gaining a pound is entirely too easy! One pound of fat equals 3,500 calories. If you eat 500 more calories than your body needs each day for a week, there's going to be a one-pound jump up on the scale come Monday morning. And those 500 extra calories can be picked up in the time it takes to grab a handful of cookies from his cupboard or have seconds at dinner just because he's still eating.

Of course, this can go the other way, too. By dropping those little noshing habits, you can drop a pound of fat a week. Just don't go under 1,200 calories per day. Your body will think it's stranded on an island and go into starvation mode—which will do the one thing you definitely don't want: slam the brakes on your metabolism. This slow-down causes the body to hold onto calories rather than burn them off. Once you start turning the metabolism down, it's hard to turn it back up. So when you start to eat normally again—no woman can eat like a bird forever!—any weight you've lost will come back quickly. So watch the extra snacks, but make sure to eat!

THE SKINNY ON SIZE

You don't need anyone to tell you when those pants start to feel tight, but there's a delicate balance between being a little bit heavier than you'd like and tipping the scales toward a slew of health problems. A general rule of thumb for finding out if your weight is on target is the body mass index (BMI); it estimates your total body fat, rather than focusing on pounds. However, this formula doesn't take into account amazing biceps; so if you work out a lot, you may skew a bit higher, as a pound of muscle has more mass than a pound of fat, but it will give you an idea if you need to drop a few pounds for your health or just maintain what you've got. According to the National Institutes of Health, a healthy BMI for a woman falls between 18.5–24.9. You are considered overweight at 25–29.9 and obese—don't you hate how that word sounds?—at 30 or higher.

Find your BMI by dividing your weight by your height in inches squared and multiplying it by 703: $(\text{weight}/[\text{height(in)}]^2) \times 703 = \text{BMI}$

For example, if you are 130 pounds and 5′4″, your math should look like this:

1. 5 feet x 12 inches = 60 inches + 4 inches = 64 (height in inches)

2. Then multiply 64 by 64 (doing the squared part first makes it easier!) to get 4,096.

3. Then divide your weight (130) by 4,096 to get .031738281.

4. Multiply .031738281 by 703, and you get a BMI of 22.31.

If your BMI is over 25, don't freak out. You can start taking better care of yourself by eating healthier and moving more, which will make a big difference in how your life unfolds. Studies have shown that dropping your weight by as little as 5 percent can lower blood pressure and cholesterol and decrease your risk for diabetes.

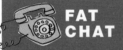

FAT CHAT REAL WOMEN WEIGH IN ON HOW HIS FOOD HABITS AFFECT THEM

"He definitely eats more often than I need to, and it is a challenge not to succumb and eat because the foods are there." —Karen, 25

"He eats whatever he pleases, and his abs are toned as ever. Believe me—it's not from the gym!" —Elena, 21

"It's so hard to have just one slice of pizza, especially when he's already had five!" —Emily, 25

"I admire his ability to eat crap and not gain weight." —Sadie, 19

"He always wants to order an appetizer, even at lunch." —Tina, 25

INSULIN AND MUFFIN TOPS

The more weight you gain now, the harder it will be to lose later. That's because extra weight—especially too much flab around the waist—can lead to insulin resistance, a condition that makes shedding extra pounds difficult.

Insulin is a storage hormone made by the pancreas that allows the body to use food as energy. Every time you eat something, the food is broken down into glucose, a form of sugar that the body uses for fuel. The glucose floats in the bloodstream until the insulin "unlocks" the cells, so they can suck in the glucose and burn it for energy—or store it as fat to use later.

When you have insulin resistance, your body doesn't respond to insulin as it should. It becomes less sensitive to the hormone, and so, in order to deal with glucose in the bloodstream—too much makes you sick—the body produces extra insulin to keep blood sugar levels stable. Because insulin is always trying to hold onto sugar and store it, too much insulin makes losing weight extremely difficult. And excess insulin will make you even hungrier, which leads to a cycle of eating more, which makes you gain more, which makes it harder to lose weight. Over time, high insulin levels can lead to type 2 diabetes, a disease that occurs when the pancreas finally becomes so tired from working overtime that it stops making enough insulin. Not only is diabetes a difficult disease to live with—it requires constant monitoring and lifestyle changes—but it can also lead to heart disease, kidney failure, and blindness. So how can you give it your best shot to stay thin and healthy? Read on.

WISE-GUY RULE

Don't try to keep up with the big boys. By eating slower than your BFB's gulp-without-chewing pace, your plate will always be occupied—which means he'll be less inclined to force-feed you any of his scraps.

THE SMART GIRL'S GUIDE TO FOOD

With all the confusion over good fats and bad fats, good carbs and bad carbs, it can be incredibly hard for any girl to know what she should be eating for a hot and healthy body. Here are some basic guidelines. Just remember: THIS IS NOT A DIET! It's just healthful eating. Diets make you feel totally restricted and screwed up, so stay away from them. Do your best to eat what is good for your body and what makes you feel strong, healthy, and gorgeous. That said, you probably shouldn't have a huge bowl of ice cream every night. But if you want to have a serving and follow these basic guidelines for the rest of the day, go for it!

Forget the pyramid. Instead of following the triangle's recommendation for getting the majority of calories from whole grains, pastas, cereals, and rice, think of your base as nonstarchy vegetables: big leafy salads, spinach, tomatoes, celery, red and green peppers, squash, broccoli, cauliflower, asparagus—the list goes on and on.

Daily dose: Eat as many veggies as you want! They're low in calories and packed with cancer- and wrinkle-fighting antioxidants. Carb-heavy veggies such as potatoes, peas, and corn should be thought of as breads rather than as veggies and should be eaten in moderation.

. . . .

Fruit is fab. Strawberries, blueberries, cherries, peaches, pears, plums, apples, melons—these are nature's sweet treats and are full of good-for-you antioxidants and other nutrients like vitamin C and fiber.

Daily dose: Aim for 3–5 servings a day. Although they're not total freebies like the wonderful world of veggies, if it's between candy and grapes, go with the grapes!

. . . .

Protein power. Whether you're a meat lover or a meat hater, protein is the building block of muscle, hair, skin, and all the cells in your body. Studies have shown it to be the most satiating of food groups, beating out both carbs and fat. Opt for lean meats, low-fat dairy, tofu, soymilk, and nuts and legumes (aka beans).

Daily dose: It depends on your size. Divide your weight in half and then subtract 10. That number indicates how many grams of protein you need each day. So if you weigh 135 pounds, you need 58 grams of this power group every 24 hours.

. . . .

Fat facts. Eating fat doesn't mean you'll be fat. The body needs some fat to maintain body heat and protect organs. The fats to avoid are saturated and trans-fats. They move through your veins like a solid block of butter, which can lead to high cholesterol levels in the body — a precursor to heart disease and stroke. The good fats are monounsaturated and polyunsaturated fats.

Daily dose: Good or bad, you still don't need very much. That's because fats are so weighty — one gram contains nine calories, which is double the number of calories in carbs and proteins. For example, a single tablespoon of oil has 120 calories! The USDA recommends that 30 percent of your daily calories come from fat, but the American Heart Association recommends that no more than 7 percent of daily calories come from saturated fat. (For a 2,000 calorie diet, that's about 16 grams.) Aim for as little trans-fat as possible — zero is best!

. . . .

Friendly fiber. Unlike carbs, fats, and protein, fiber cannot be absorbed by the body. Fiber passes through your system — the stomach, small intestine, and finally, the colon — unchanged. Think of it as a big, clean sweep for the body: While it's moving through the digestive system, fiber makes you feel full, detoxifies the body, and lowers the risk of high cholesterol, heart disease, and diabetes. And it keeps things moving in the bathroom, too, which can prevent nasty things like hemorrhoids or irritable bowel syndrome (IBS).

bfb real-life story

Your BF doesn't have to be fat in order to make it easy for you to gain weight. Avantika, 28, found out that even though her man is slim and healthy, he can still weigh her down if she's not careful.

"He eats constantly," says Avantika, who has been with her now-fiancé for the past three years. "He can't go more than one hour without getting hungry for another snack or meal." Her soon-to-be hubby is also incredibly fit and exercises almost daily, which means he eats as much as he wants, as often as he wants, without gaining weight. "I have to remind myself that, even though I work out, I have nowhere near the caloric requirements that he does," says Avantika, recalling her initial five-pound gain when they first started dating.

In order to stay slim, she now shares meals with him when they go out. She knows he'll eat more than half. "I also had to lay down some ground rules about which snacks are not allowed in the house," she says. "I don't allow ice cream except for special occasions. Otherwise, he'll buy a huge container and eat some every night while I look on jealously or break down and eat unnecessary dessert as well!"

Daily dose: Women need about 25 grams of fiber daily (BFBs should have about 38 grams). Most Americans get only 10–15 grams of fiber per day, which is not enough for optimal health. But if you reach for lots of fruits (apples, pears), veggies (artichokes, cucumbers, broccoli), and whole grains (brown rice, oats, wheat bread), you'll meet that goal in no time.

. . . .

Refrain from refined. White bread, white rice, pasta, sugary cereals, and anything made with white flour are refined carbohydrates. This means they started out as a grain—either wheat, rice, barley, or corn—but have had the fiber (the bran and the germ—the part that's really good for you!) removed. Because there isn't any—or very little—fiber to slow down how fast they're digested, the body quickly turns them to sugar, thus shooting up blood sugar and insulin levels.

Daily dose: This depends on your activity level. The more you're burning, the more carbs you can eat without care. In general, try to eat as few of these as possible, and when you do reach for carbs, go with the unrefined ones, like whole-wheat pasta, brown rice, brown breads, and oats. They'll digest more slowly.

. . . .

Sugar sucks. This sweetie is a big cause of added pounds. It's as refined a carb as you can get, so it raises blood sugar levels and causes the body to produce more insulin. And the amount of nutrition it adds to your diet is a big fat zero—there's nothing in sugar but calories.

Daily dose: It's hard to avoid, but you want to eat as little sugar as possible. The 2005 Dietary Guidelines for Americans leave room for only 8 teaspoons of the sweet stuff per day—which is less than the amount in a regular 12-ounce can of Coke! That doesn't mean never having a few Sour Patch Kids if they're your fave, but don't eat them everyday for lunch, either.

Keep it real. In a world full of the artificial—from noses to boobs to food—it's easy to get caught up in the whole "sugar-free, calorie-free" nonsense. But artificial sweeteners aren't the little magic freebies you may think they are. Researchers warn that they can actually make you *gain* weight. A study published in the American Psychological Association's *Behavioral Neuroscience* journal found that rats given sugar substitutes ate more and gained more weight than those that ate—get this—real, honest-to-goodness sugar. And, unfortunately, you don't need to consume pounds of the stuff to feel the adverse effects. Research shows that drinking just one can of diet soda a day can cause weight gain.

Daily dose: So if you're a regular diet soda guzzler, put the can, er, two-liter bottle, down and reach for water, seltzer, or unsweetened iced tea instead. Hold on—this doesn't mean you have to give up a sweet tooth to stay thin. See chapter 8 for other natural alternatives to sugar and these chemically-produced white powders.

BFB FINAL THOUGHT

Sometimes you have to let go of the giant bag of movie theater popcorn to get what you really want.

I know that movie-theater popcorn is bad for me. Still, it takes very little for my BFB to convince me that we need a jumbo-sized bag. Of course, the second the lights dim, I immediately start the nonstop hand-to-mouth motion that can lead to only one thing: an empty bag and a stomach too full to find the prospect of a real dinner one bit enticing. But as my BFB reaches over to grab another handful, our fingers brush about halfway down the greasy bag. And I realize, what I really want to be holding is not to be found within the confines of a paper bag. What I really want to be holding is his hand.

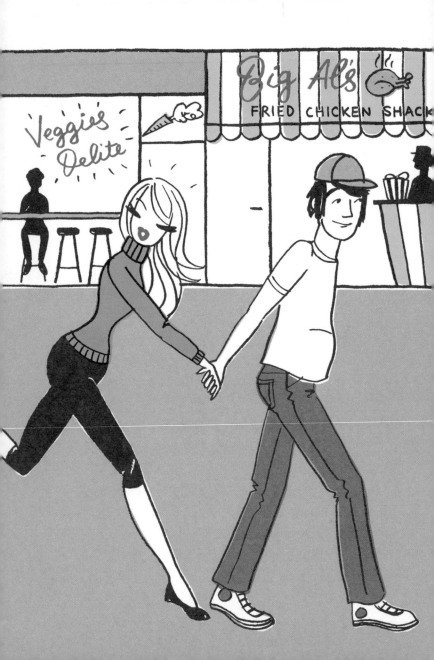

CHAPTER 4

EATING OUT

It's Friday night, and I'm ready to kill the sadist who decided to take a cheesecake—one of the most calorie-rich desserts ever created—and fry it. Actually dip it in hot, greasy fat, and dust it with an irresistible coating.

What's worse is that if this dirty bomb of diet self-control ends up on the table, I know I won't stop until I'm scraping the last bit of melted ice cream from the dish. "Dessert?" the waitress asks, her voice so syrupy-sweet you'd think she was offering a multivitamin instead of coronary disease on a plate. I picture the hours of sweat I'll have to log at the gym as the order rolls off my BFB's tongue, his face so happy I can almost see his invisible tail wagging. "I can't wait," he tells me.

It wasn't until my jeans were snug that I realized I was going to need some serious dining-out defenses. These going-out guidelines will allow you to eat, drink and look forward to table time with your honey—without taking home unwanted pounds.

PICKING THE PLACE

Some nights—when your guy has a big night out planned or you're meeting up with friends—you won't have a say in where you end up. But if it's an average night out, put some thought into your dining destination. You'll be surprised at the difference in your waistline.

Take a hint. If there's a blinking neon sign heralding the name "F.A.T.S." (this is an actual restaurant in New York City), rethink stepping foot in the front door.

Shake things up. If you eat until you can no longer breathe every time you and your sweetheart hit the local chain, try a new cuisine. Chinese, Japanese, seafood, and Mediterranean joints have tons of healthy menu options. Look for dishes that are packed with colorful, yummy veggies and avoid anything that is breaded or fried.

Do some sleuthing. Almost all restaurants have menus online, and many big chains even have nutritional info so you can check out the potential muffin-top factor beforehand. Walk in knowing you want the veggie stir-fry, and you won't be as dissuaded by your BFB when he orders mac and cheese.

Compromise. Sure, you won't be able to pick the place every night, but if you make little compromises with your sweetie—he can pick the movie if you can pick the restaurant—you won't be doomed to eat at the greasy spoon down the road or the sports bar that specializes in deep-fried foods every time you dine out.

Find strength in numbers. If you are mutual friends with another couple, conspire with your girlfriend to dine at a new, healthier restaurant. It will be easier to convince your men to agree to go if they know their buddy is being dragged along as well.

DRESS UP!

Whether you're heading to the same neighborhood spot you've been to a million times or you're just heading out to meet your man at the local diner for a late-night nosh, slipping into those totally hot new jeans or that daring little low-cut top will help you avoid overdoing it once you pull up to the table. Put on something that makes you feel totally gorgeous, even if it's as simple as a pair of heels or a spritz of your favorite perfume. Sure, your guy will appreciate the sexy surprise, but this is for you. The better you feel in your skin, the more you'll want to put something good in your body. And when you can actually see your figure instead of hiding it beneath a sweatshirt, you'll be a lot less inclined to polish off your boy's leftover onion rings.

RAVENOUS IS RISKY

Whatever you do, don't go starving. Hungry—as in, you had lunch and it's now a few hours later—is fine. But if you hit the table famished enough to eat the raspberry lip gloss you just slicked on, the caloric weight of today's appetizers—not to mention the breadbasket—could easily wipe out your recommended daily allotment before you even see your entrée.

So be smart. Enjoy your day leading up to dinner. Have a normal breakfast, a lighter lunch, and grab an apple or string cheese an hour or so before dinner. Not only will you avoid blowing your day on the appetizer, but you'll have a saner approach to the menu. When you're starving and your blood sugar is low, you won't end up ordering what's good for you.

WISE-GUY RULE

Take one for the team and eat at whatever grease dispenser is showing Monday Night Football. This will give you bargaining power over where you chow down Tuesday through Sunday. No clue what to order? Go with a burger, forgo the cheese (you'll save more than 100 calories), eat only half the roll, and sub the fries for a baked potato or a side salad (just use the dressing sparingly or go for a fat-free balsamic vinaigrette). No damage done, and you've got the rest of the week to twist his arm into trying that new sushi place you've been dying to check out!

QUICK PICKS

No matter what the cuisine, you can always find a healthy dish. Next time you're out, try one of these yummy, better-for-your-bod alternatives.

American: If they have a low-cal or Weight Watchers menu, go with that—they're surprisingly delish! If not, pick grilled chicken over fried and a side salad instead of fries.

Chinese: Chicken and broccoli, shrimp and snow peas, and spicy chicken and string beans are all packed with protein and low in fat and carbs. Keep your hand away from the bowl of those fried crunchy noodles and sip tea instead.

Diner: Avoid the mayo-doused chicken and tuna salad, and cut fat and calories in omelets by asking for egg whites, dry whole-wheat toast, and a side of fruit instead of hash browns.

Indian: Stick to baked tandoori (chicken marinated in yogurt), chicken masala (chicken chunks spiced with curry), and veggie-based dishes. Beware of the bread: Naan, chapati, and roti breads are usually fried or brushed with butter.

Italian: Stay away from fat-laden alfredo and stuffed-cheese dishes; try the minestrone soup, tomato and moz-zarella, or pasta with tomato-based sauces. Ask if breaded dishes, such as eggplant and chicken parmigiana, can be baked instead of fried.

Mediterranean: Grilled shrimp, beautifully tossed salads, light vinaigrettes, fresh fruit, grilled tuna, chicken pita sandwiches . . . there are tons of diet-friendly options here. Save the carb-heavy pasta dishes for another night.

Mexican: Swap out those refried beans—they're almost always made with lard—for low-fat black or pinto beans, and stick to chicken fajitas instead of the cheese-filled enchiladas. Order all sour cream, guacamole, and cheese on the side, but enjoy as much salsa and hot sauce as you want.

Pub fare: Go with broth-based soups, grilled chicken, pot roast—sans gravy—or salad with dressing on the side. Portions are usually double what you need, so sit close to your honey and share. Avoid the apps; you'll be hard-pressed to find one that isn't deep-fried or loaded with calories.

Seafood: There are lots of healthy picks from under the sea. Fish is chockfull of healthy omega-3 fatty acids, and shrimp, clams, oysters, and crabs are—as long as they're not deep-fried—full of low-fat protein. Opt for baked or broiled entrées and squirt on lemon for flavor in place of butter or high-fat tartar sauce.

Sushi: Skip the fried tempura roll to save fat and calories and opt for a spicy tuna or California roll instead. If your BFB begs for an appetizer, munch on yummy but healthy edamame—low-fat soybeans full of protein and fiber.

BUT I HATE VEGGIES!

OK, so not every girl is gonna be gaga over a big, green salad. But that doesn't mean you have to soak up thousands of calories on a night out, either. If you'll only be happy with the penne alla vodka, then get it. Just add a few tummy-taming tweaks. Ask for whole-wheat pasta and request that the chef toss in some grilled chicken. Then you'll be getting the dish you love, but with healthier carbs and a good dose of satiating protein. Eat half, have it boxed, and then focus on slowly nursing a glass of red wine. (For savvier menu skills, see "Made to Order," page 56.)

---

bfb real-life story

Remember when you picked at your food like a bird on your first date, too afraid you'd end up with something on your face to really enjoy the meal? Ha! Not anymore! Kelly, 25, went from five-bites-and-I'm-done to holy crap, I'm too full to budge!

"Jamie and I had been dating for about eight months and it was our first Christmas together," says Kelly. "We had a party to go to that evening, but he was hungry so we went out for Mexican. After an appetizer (I never ordered them before, but now I share them with Jamie), a taco, burrito, enchilada, and something that was basically a huge plate of cheese, by the time we got to the party, we were miserable. We just sat on the couch the entire night and didn't move!"

MADE TO ORDER

Speaking up can make a huge difference in slimming down. Go ahead and be picky when placing your order. Your guy will think it's cute—or he'll love to tease you about it. Either way, it's a great excuse to banter back and forth and teach him a little Health 101 while you're at it. Besides, what guy doesn't love a girl who knows what she wants?

TEN REQUESTS TO ADD TO YOUR REGULAR DINING REPERTOIRE

1. **Dressing on the side**
2. **Grilled instead of fried**
3. **Steamed, not sautéed**
4. **Hold the bacon, butter, or sour cream** (or ask for them on the side)
5. **Easy on the sauce**
6. **Dry toast, jelly on the side**
7. **Egg whites**
8. **A baked potato instead of fries**—or, better yet, a side salad with low-fat or nonfat dressing
9. **Light on the mayo**, or fat-free mustard instead
10. **Don't butter the hamburger bun**

SLIM SECRET

While your date debates over what to order, ask the waiter for a glass of water. Make it your goal to finish it before the plates hit the table. It will fill you up and help ensure you're not eating when you're actually just parched.

TUBBY TERMS
- Au gratin
- Battered
- Béarnaise
- Breaded
- Buttered
- Cheesy
- Cream(y)
- Crispy
- Deep-fried
- Fried
- Pan-fried
- Rich
- Sautéed
- White sauce

WAIST-FRIENDLY WORDS
- Baked
- Braised
- Cajun
- Grilled
- Marinated
- Poached
- Seared
- Slow-cooked
- Spicy
- Steamed
- Tomato-based

FAST-FOOD FIXES

The French fry smell is wafting in the air, your BFB is ticking off his list of biggie everything, and you've got less than a minute to order. Don't crack under pressure! Here are some tips and tricks for what to choose when your BFB insists on rolling through the drive-thru.

TACO BELL

Best bets: Fresco Ranchero Chicken Soft Taco or Fresco Grilled Steak Soft Taco. They're fewer than 200 calories each and have only 4.5 grams of fat. On the other hand, they have more than 10 grams of hunger-staving protein.

Avoid: The salads. Surprise! The Fiesta Taco Salad clocks in at more than 800 calories. If you're dying to go "green," lose the fried shell and you'll save almost 400 calories.

Helpful hint: Ditch the side of sour cream (80 calories) and the guacamole (70 calories), and go with the salsa (it has only 15!).

BURGER KING

Best bets: The Tendergrill Chicken Garden Salad or a plain ol' hamburger. The salad has only 240 calories, 9 grams of fat, 8 grams of carbs — 4 of which are fiber —

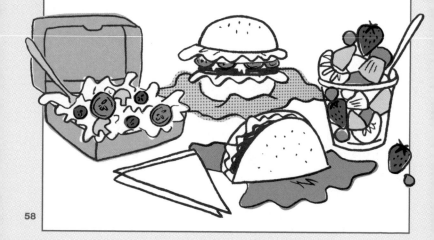

and more than 30 grams of protein. (Use half the packet of light Italian dressing or the fat-free ranch dressing and you'll have a filling lunch for an even 300 calories.) The burger, although not as healthy, still weighs in just under 300 calories. But if you add cheese, tack on an extra 50.

Avoid: Even a bite of his lunch, especially if it's the BK Quad Stacker (1,010 calories) or the Triple Whopper Sandwich with cheese (almost a day's worth of calories: 1,250).

Helpful hint: If you know you're gonna eat a few of his fries, ask for a knife and a fork and order that burger bunless. They will package it in a cute container with a little lettuce and tomato, sans carb-filled bun.

ARBY'S

Best bets: Martha's Vineyard Salad (272 calories) or the Kid's Meal Junior Roast Beef Sandwich (273 calories). Ask for the kid's fruit cup (only 34 calories!) for a sweet ending.

Avoid: Popcorn chicken—a large has more than 500 calories. Which means having a few pieces can easily equal a 100-calorie splurge . . . and that's without any of the fatty dipping sauces!

Helpful hint: From grilled chicken to roast beef, this place puts mayo on almost everything. Ask them to hold it and you'll save about 100 calories.

MCDONALD'S

Best bets: Any of the salads are pretty good, as long as you ask for grilled chicken and one of the low-fat dressings. If you want beef, stay basic. A hamburger is 250 calories (get the cheeseburger, and you'll ratchet it up to 300). If you want an ice cream hit, go with the vanilla cone: it's a doable 150.

Avoid: Besides the big burgers, stay away from the Deluxe Breakfast (it'll start your morning at 1,080 calories — and that's without syrup or margarine). An M&M McFlurry will cost you more than 600 calories, and a Triple Thick Shake will triple the size of your thighs in no time — a 16-ounce chocolate swirls in at 580 calories.

Helpful hint: At McDonald's, the word *premium* doesn't mean better for you, it just means bigger! The Premium Grilled Chicken Classic Sandwich is 420 calories — 60 more than the crispy McChicken.

WENDY'S

Best bets: The Mandarin Chicken Salad is only 170 calories . . . until you add the roasted almonds and crispy noodles, which bring it close to 400. Drizzle on the Oriental sesame dressing and you'll rack it up to more than 500 calories. So, swap the dressing for the reduced-fat creamy ranch, use half the packet (45 calories), and enjoy with half the crispy noodles and half the almonds;

you'll bring it back down to a reasonable 300. Or go with the small chili (220 calories, 17 grams of protein, and 5 grams of fiber) and the reduced-fat milk (120 calories) for a total of 340 protein-packed calories.

Avoid: The Triple with Everything and Cheese. At 980 calories, that's triple what any girl needs for lunch, especially if you tack on a few fries and a drink!

Helpful hint: Don't fall for the "small" theory here. Small fries and a small chocolate Frosty are gonna cost you more than a hefty 300 calories each.

SUBWAY

Best bets: Six- or four-inch basic sandwiches, like turkey or ham, since they have less than 300 calories each. The salads are super low in calories (the highest comes in at 280). Just go with oil and vinegar or the fat-free dressing.

Avoid: The six-inch Meatball Marinara and Chicken & Bacon Ranch have almost 600 calories each, and the six-inch tuna is still heavy at 530.

Helpful hint: If you're really hungry, stick with a six-inch and ask for double meat instead of filling up with a foot-long full of bread or wasting calories on a bag of chips. If you really want those chips, compromise by ordering a salad or a four-incher to cut down on carbs.

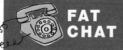

FAT CHAT

TIPS AND TRICKS ON DINING OUT FROM REAL WOMEN LIKE YOU

"Talk! The meal goes slower and you'll eat less." —Carly, 21

"The hardest part about eating out is not polishing off my plate! I have to always remind myself to halve the portion and place it directly into a doggie bag." —Elena, 21

"I try to ask myself beforehand, 'What do I feel like tonight? Do I really want something fattening or unhealthy?' Sometimes the answer is 'yes,' and I go with it. But if I feel like eating light I try to recognize that and remind myself when I'm ordering." —Jane, 24

"After eating one piece, push the bread basket to his side of the table and don't complain when he leans over and steals from your plate!" —Carly, 21

"I usually have a salad before I go out to curb my appetite." —Nicole, 18

"Stick with your healthy habits and don't let your man convince you that a steak, potato, bread, and some cheesecake aren't that bad for you. If you had bread at breakfast or lunch, skip it at dinner." —Jammie, 26

JUST A TASTE

Sharing can be fun, but don't think a nibble of this and a taste of that goes unnoticed. Even if you're not counting calories, your body is. Watch out for these calorie calamities.

- Three pieces of fried cheese with marinara sauce: more than 400 calories and 29 grams of fat
- Three boneless buffalo wings with bleu cheese: almost 400 calories and 30 grams of fat

- Only one-fifth of an onion blossom with dipping sauce: almost 600 calories and 40 grams of fat
- Half a basket of nacho chips with salsa: 240 calories and 18 grams of fat
- A quarter of the fries that come with his burger: more than 100 calories and almost 7 grams of fat
- Half a slice of cheesecake: almost 400 calories and 20 grams of fat

SIP SMART

Sitting with your boy at the bar or romantically sharing a tall, frosty milkshake at the diner can be a lot of fun. But if you don't want to derail your waist-watching work in a single gulp, be careful about what's in your cup. Many drinks are filled with hidden calories, and because there's no chewing involved, you don't fill up or feel full.

Cream = calories. Yeah, those frozen mudslides and ice cream-swirled milkshakes on the next table over look unbelievable, but don't let him talk you into sharing one! It would take more than an hour on the treadmill to burn off their whopping caloric weight.

Go light. If you want to enjoy a cold beer without adding to your belly, opt for the lower-cal, low-carb alternatives. You'll save about 50 calories per bottle by downgrading to Miller Lite, Amstel Light, Bud Light, or Michelob Ultra.

Fruit can be fattening. Many bars use juices that are filled with sugary syrups. Lighten up a cranberry and vodka by asking for seltzer, vodka, and just a splash of cranberry. You'll cut sugar and calories and add lots of refreshing bubbles. This trick works great with any juice-flavored beverage.

Keep tabs on your tab. Even hard alcohol counts: The average shot has between 50 and 80 calories! And watch how quickly you're emptying that glass. The more buzzed you become, the less you'll care about watching what you're eating—and drinking!

Rethink that H2O. If plain old *agua* doesn't do it for you, add a spritz of lemon or lime. Not only will you get a boost of refreshing citrus flavor, you'll score some immune-building vitamin C while you're at it. And if you're craving the bubbly goodness of soda, try seltzer. It has zero calories and chemicals but all the fizz you're after.

Say goodbye to sugar. This sweet stuff is the white devil to dieters. It's loaded with calories and has zero nutritional value. Avoid sugar-saturated mixed drinks like daiquiris and margaritas—which can easily pack more than 500 calories—and opt for a glass of wine or light beer.

Spice things up. Try a Bloody Mary for a spicy kick—and some heart-healthy veggies. Go virgin and you'll cut the calories almost in half.

Watch that wine. Dessert wines have almost double the

calories of the drier whites or reds, which already tote between 70 and 80 calories per glass. So enjoy a serving with your meal, but steer clear of after-dinner bottles.

BFB FINAL THOUGHT

Forget the mints . . . and whatever else is by the register.

Some rocket scientist who owns a diner on Long Island must have thought to himself one day: "You know what I'm going to do? I'm going to put free cookies on a platter for people to take when they walk out." That or the Gods of Good Nutrition were testing me once again. On this particular dining excursion, I avoid dessert— sometimes a check dropped too early works in a girl's favor—and head to the bathroom (all that water has to go somewhere!) while my BFB heads to the counter to pay the check. I return to find him holding the front door for me, cookie crumbs on his cheek, the smell of sugar on his breath, a dumb smile on his face, and, nestled into his fist, two extra cookies for the road. "I got you one," he tells me. If only he wasn't so damn adorable, with his mussed-up hair and corduroy jacket; I swear I'd be 15 pounds lighter. Thankfully, it's one of those bland-tasting, grandma's-biscuits-in-a-tin-can kinds of sugar cookies, so I ignore the offer and lean up and give him a kiss instead. Sometimes, that's the sweetest ending I need.

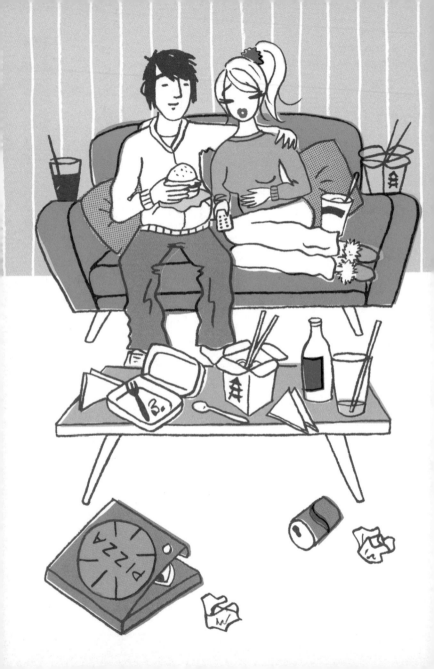

CHAPTER 5

ORDERING IN

The amount of fat and calories swarming around in my belly must be off the charts. I have just consumed half of an extra-crispy, extra-melty pizza. Half. As in, three times the amount I should have eaten.

My BFB told me he was ordering a thin-crust pie, and in a weak moment—I'd like to blame it on coupons and a too-comfy pair of sweatpants—I dumbly agreed. I allowed myself to be swayed by the word "thin," thinking it meant there would be less dough and that it had to be the most carb-conscious pizza purveyed by this obesity-friendly vendor. But "somehow"—as in, he didn't actually order a thin-crust pizza but went with some "special" pizza they had a "great deal on"—what showed up could never be classified by a word remotely close to "thin." When the disaster of a pie arrived, my BFB slid the warm, fragrant box onto the coffee table and dramatically threw open the top. We stood side by side, looking down at our delivered dinner.

"Awesome!" He reached for a slice, digging in as I stood by silently.

"It looks so greasy," I said, frowning as I noticed the fatty puddles pooling on top of the cheesy topping.

"Well, you got half with green peppers," my boyfriend with the amazing memory so kindly reminded me. "No way am I touching that." I grabbed a few napkins and dabbed at a slice, sopping up whatever fat I could.

"Come on, it's good!" He waited for me to take a taste like a gang member waiting for a newbie to take her first hit.

Damn. It was good. "OK," I admitted. "It's edible."

And then, everything went hazy. All I remember is that we were watching *Curb Your Enthusiasm,* and when I looked up, there was nothing left but the greasy wax paper and a few gobs of totally unappetizing cheese staring back at me accusingly.

"I feel ill," I tell my accomplice, who is happily spread out on the other end of the couch.

"I can't believe you ate Domino's with me." He's smiling, totally content.

"I know," I groan. "Me neither."

"That was awesome. Half a pie! You never used to eat this stuff. I'm so proud of you."

"Stop, stop talking about it. I don't want to think about it." I groan and gingerly readjust my position on the couch, so as not to disturb my protruding paunch.

"We still have more coupons. . . . "

I playfully whack him with a pillow.

As we settle down for another round of Larry David foolery, my mind floats back to his previous comment. What had just happened? This wasn't the first time I had gone overboard on takeout. Just last week I'd housed close to half of his General Tso's—on top of my own pint of shrimp and veggies.

In college, when everything was new and sparkly, and I was totally on good behavior diet-wise—I would've never okayed a Domino's dinner. I would've picked up a salad ahead of time or ordered steamed chicken and veggies from the Chinese spot on the corner, even if he ordered a cheese-filled, flour-heavy stromboli or a basket of wings from the grease pit across the street.

I had simply gotten lazy. It's easy to do when you're already in sweats and as happy as can be curled up next to the boy who finds you hot even when you have spinach in your teeth. But I knew there were plenty of easy ways to enjoy our takeout nights and not end up immobile and stuffed to capacity.

Here's how to enjoy your night without loading up during lounge time.

GROUND RULES

Eating in presents challenges entirely different from eating out. Although you still have to make smart choices when placing your order (see page 56 for sneaky ways to cut calories from your favorite dishes and page 57 for red-flag words to avoid when ordering), it's a whole 'nother ball game when you're surrounded by comfy pillows, elastic waistbands, and the TV.

These ideas and sneaky little tricks will keep you from chowing down until you feel like a verifiable couch potato, which means you'll still be interested in what's really the most fun about staying in: impromptu makeout sessions!

Mix up menus. If where you order depends on which menus were slipped under the door, it's time to put some thought into it. Try not to wait until the eleventh hour—that moment when you're drooling and famished enough to eat the last stale bits of cereal your BFB has stashed in his cupboard before the food arrives. Next time you dine out and are able to find something tasty and relatively good for you, grab a menu as you head out the door. They just might have delivery service.

On the Web, Menupages.com has a wonderful little category called "health food." Check out these restaurants' menus, and see if there are any in your area that will bring healthier takeout to your door.

Don't be threatened by minimum orders. When you're sticking to your guns (and your waistline) and ordering from a spot different than your sweetie's for a more healthful option, there's nothing more annoying than being three bucks under the delivery minimum. Rather than caving in and ordering an appetizer or a second dish you don't really want or need, add on a few bottles of water or another low-cal beverage to tip the scales in your favor.

Be daring. It can be a little risky to try an entirely new cuisine when you're spending the cash for a night out, but a night in is the perfect time to try something new. Thai, Indian, Mediterranean—there is so much more than your go-to pizza joint. And, if you don't end up liking it, grab a healthy frozen dinner from the freezer.

Use the fridge. Don't forget, you have an entire arsenal of condiments at your disposal to tweak and add flavor to any dish. When in doubt, request things dry or with no added salt. They don't have low-fat dressing? Who cares?! Use your favorite low-cal balsamic vinaigrette. They sent packets of soy sauce with enough sodium to fill the Dead Sea? Grab the low-sodium bottle hiding out behind the ketchup.

Make the call. Relinquishing the phone to him means trusting him to convey all of those specific requests (e.g., dressing on the side, without cheese, hold the bacon, no mayo). So make the call and get what you really want.

DON'T BE A BOOB TUBE

There's something fabulously mind-numbing about chilling out in front of the TV. But if you're trying to corral calorie-binges on the couch, autopilot munchies are detrimental to your waistline. If you can, enjoy your takeout with your BFB before turning on the tube. You'll eat slower, which will allow your body to register that you are, in fact, no longer starving to death.

If munching mindlessly is too tempting to pass up, do not, on penalty of a bigger pair of pants, bring an entire bag, box, or carton with you to the couch. If it's there, you will eat it . . . and eat it . . . and eat it . . . until it is gone. Research shows that the more people are served, the more they will eat. So instead of arranging the entire spread on the coffee table mere inches away from you, drop off the boxes in the kitchen and fix a plate. Just make it a small one: Research shows that the smaller the dish—and utensils—the less you'll eat. Opt for a small fork or spoon and a salad plate or bowl. If you're still truly hungry, you can always go back for more.

Then, before you sit down, dim the lights, light some candles—yummy vanilla is best; It may satisfy your after-dinner sweet tooth without any calories! And when your plate is empty, snuggle and enjoy the show. You'll be less inclined to get up from a horizontal position for seconds . . . especially if he's lying next to you.

MAKE YOUR OWN APPETIZERS

If you can't avoid the bread basket when eating out, eating in means you don't have to down hundreds of calories before the main meal arrives. Instead of choosing something from the calorie-laden menu—if your BFB protests, point out that whatever you order won't truly be an app since it will arrive at the same time as the food anyway—grab one of the following from the fridge.

Apples and peanut butter: Thinly slice two green apples and arrange them on a plate with a tablespoon of peanut butter. You're getting fruit and some hunger-staving healthy fats and protein.

Baby carrots and low-fat dressing: This crunchy snack will abate some of that hunger while providing healthy-but-filling fiber and a serving or two of veggies— something you may be in need of if you're opting for a dinner of pizza and beer!

High-fiber tortillas and low-fat hummus: Even BFBs love this one! Pull apart the tortillas and dip little pieces into the low-fat hummus and you'll score lots of filling fiber. Better yet, pair the hummus with celery and baby carrots.

Low-fat French onion soup: Grab a prepared container or a can from the grocery store. All you have to do is heat it, toss in a few croutons or half-slice of whole grain bread, and melt a thin slice of mozzarella over the top (just pop it in the microwave for about a minute). And if you really want to watch calories (or feel ultra lazy) just sip the broth—it tastes almost as good sans toppings.

Olives and pickles: Create your own little antipasto plate. Olives are full of good-for-you fats, and pickles are just cucumbers dressed up for a party. You'll avoid the carb overload in a bag of chips and even sneak some veggies into your boy. (Who thinks of a pickle as a veggie?)

Salsa and baked corn chips: Salsa is nothing but good for you: it's full of veggies and super low in calories and fat. Break the chips into pieces so you get more dip for your dough while loading up on veggies and eating fewer chips.

STOP NIBBLING AFTER YOU'RE FULL

With unlimited access to the fridge, it can be all too easy to find yourself wandering back into the kitchen for a bite between commercials—especially when your BFB wants to share a late-night snack. So as soon as you finish eating, clear away leftovers, pop a piece of gum, or brush your teeth. Then get your hands busy. Whether that means holding his, warming them around a hot mug of tea, trading shoulder rubs, or grabbing a deck of cards and playing your favorite game between commercials, find something that will get your mind off noshing. Not only will it eliminate a huge chunk of extra calories, but you'll feel better when you crawl into bed without a bulging belly.

> ### bfb real-life story
>
> *Carrie, 30, has gained more than 20 pounds since moving in with her man, and she finds ordering takeout one of her biggest binging obstacles.*
>
> "It's virtually impossible to order healthful, low-fat takeout," she says. "He wants sesame chicken and pizza, and 'Oh, look! There's free dessert pizza!' Damn the dessert pizza!" Though she cooks as often as possible, ordering in is almost always ugly.
>
> To watch her waistline, she now makes the extra effort to pick up healthier food for nights on the couch—even if it means driving to pick it up. "Somewhere I can get soup or a veggie plate. Or," she says, laughing, "if we order pizza, I'll take out two pieces for myself, close the box, hand it to him, and tell him not to let me eat any more!"

KEEP THE NIGHT ROCKIN'

If romance is on the menu—and, seriously, why shouldn't it be?—don't eat until you can't move. Not only will it keep you from feeling attractive, but eating too much or too many carbs can make you feel sleepy rather than sexy. So if you're in the mood for a romp, don't ruin it; opt for a salad with grilled chicken or chicken and string beans.

Try not to hold out all day for a big meal at night. If you eat smaller meals throughout the day, including a less-than-large dinner, you'll be a lot more interested in him! Though it's tempting to chopstick-shovel the rest of the rice, there's nothing better than snuggling up with your honey for something even sweeter than dessert!

PIZZA, AGAIN?

Even if you had pizza only occasionally before shacking up with your hottie, chances are you're seeing a whole lot more of this basic Italian standby. Pizza might as well be the fifth food group, the way BFBs scarf it down! And, although it's never a super low-cal option, it doesn't have to derail you.

Fraction facts. Most of the time, pies are cut into eighths. So, one slice of a medium pizza is smaller than one slice of a large pizza, and therefore it has fewer calories—sometimes nearly 200 fewer calories! So keep in mind that two slices of a medium pie might be doable, but one slice of a large should be dinner.

Topping truths. Cheese, sausage, and pepperoni are the toppings BFBs usually prefer to anything green, but every topping adds to the pig-out probability (except, of course, those valiant veggies). One large slice of Pizza Hut's Veggie Lover's pan pizza has 40 fewer calories than a slice of their basic pan pizza with cheese. Lesson learned: The more veggies on there, the less room for cheese and any other fatty foods.

Crust confessions. The type of floury goodness that makes up the base makes a big difference in your waistline. Although you should check online for nutrition info (these menus change constantly), the basic rule of thumb is this: Thin-crust is best; pan pizza is the worst. It's thicker, greasier, and crammed with about 100 calories more per slice than any thin-crust version.

Super specials. Crispy, melty, supreme, ultimate—all words to steer clear of when ordering. No matter how new or discounted they may be, they'll add up to hundreds of additional calories per slice. You'll take an already hefty 400-calorie large pepperoni slice from Pizza Hut and rack it up to 530 for a Meat Lover's of the same size. So stick to the basics and keep pizza simple.

Ditch dessert. Unless there's a party going on and 10 people will each have a bite or two, don't even bring these pizza imposters into the house. A Cinna Swirl Sweetreat from Papa John's has 780 calories and 28 grams of fat—10 of which are the heart-clogging saturated kind. Domino's OREO Dessert Pizza has 960 calories and 32 grams of fat. And the Cinnamon Sticks from Pizza Hut aren't much better: two (with icing) will set you back almost 400 calories and 5 grams of fat.

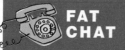

"When eating carbs for dinner, avoid fried or breaded appetizers." —Carly, 21

"If it's pizza, forgo the crust or order a thin-crust. If it's Chinese, order food with a good amount of vegetables over brown rice—and no MSG!" —Molly, 21

"I try to order as healthy as I can for myself, so if I steal a few bites of his food, I've at least gotten some nutrition first. Then, I try to think about how happy I'll be tomorrow if I stop eating now and save my leftovers for lunch the next day!" —Emily, 25

BFB FINAL THOUGHT

The gods must have a sense of humor when it comes to BFBs—that, or he's one himself!

I reach my chopsticks over to his sesame chicken and grab a wonderfully gooey, sugary-sweet piece. I pop it in my mouth even though I've been full for the past 10 minutes. He's ordered about three more entrées than we'd ever really need, and I've spent much more time helping him make a dent in those dishes than working on my pint of veggies.

"Okay, that's it. I'm totally full," I announce.

"Good," he teases me, as I reach for another crispy noodle. "I thought you were going to eat all my General Tso's."

I realize I'm eating for no other reason than because the food's staring me in the face, so I quickly roll up the bag. I chuck a fortune cookie at him.

"You are awful. Like you didn't have enough to eat."

He cracks open his fortune cookie and smirks.

"What?" I ask him. "What does it say?"

He passes the tiny little slip to me.

May you always have a good appetite.

Great. Thanks, Chinese-food gods. That's just what he needs.

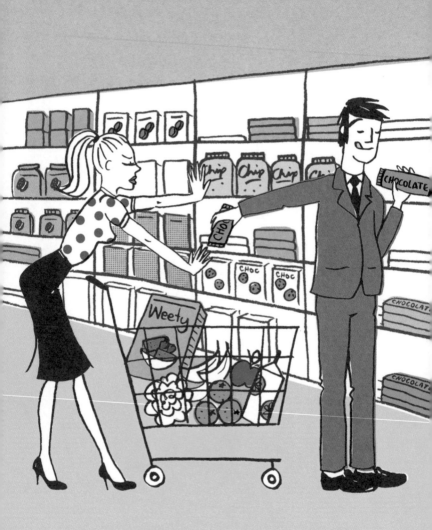

CHAPTER 6

THE
GROCERY STORE

"What about this one?" I tug on my BFB's hand and nod toward the low-fat frozen yogurt. He looks through the fogged windows and frowns.

"Raspberry? That's not ice cream. That's fruit."

He pulls me a few steps down the aisle and stops short in front of the Ben & Jerry's. He reaches in, plucks an all-too-tempting container off the shelf, and hands me the Coffee Heath Bar Crunch. I spin the carton around. "There's almost 1,200 calories in this thing. And 72 grams of fat."

He takes it back and shrugs, unconcerned. "I'm gonna get it. You know you'll want some later."

I eye the frozen dessert warily and toss a box of low-cal Fudgesicles on top, hoping I'll forget the Ben & Jerry's is even there.

The grocery store is one of your biggest battle zones. What goes into that cart has a huge probability of making its way into your mouth. Here's what to buy, when to shop, and how to keep your cart from looking like a frat boy filled it—even when he's shopping with you.

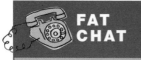

FAT CHAT

TIPS FOR THE STORE FROM REAL WOMEN LIKE YOU

"Don't let him shop! He buys Doritos and I can't have them in the house because I'll eat the entire bag." —Jill, 28

"Run through the junk food aisle. Tell him to get in the cart and push him through it!" —Lindsey, 21

"It's okay to ask the person if they really need it, or want it. And never go grocery shopping hungry or while PMSing . . . Girls really don't need an entire bag of Reese's Peanut Butter Cups!" —Molly, 21

"Keep him away from the ice cream. If there's a sale on it, he goes crazy and buys five different kinds—and when ice cream is in the house I MUST eat it!" —Emily, 25

"Separate carts or don't go at the same time!" —Jasmine, 21

"I go shopping with him at healthier supermarkets like Whole Foods and Trader Joe's. Food markets like these tend to have healthier food. At least the snacks don't have tons of artificial ingredients and preservatives." —Elena, 21

MAP YOUR MARKET

If only you could attach a little GPS to the cart that would shout out dietary directions like "Go left for veggies," and "Stop, make U-turn to avoid snack aisle." Since that's not possible, it's necessary to know the aisles as well as you know the Hollywood gossip. Otherwise, you'll end up wandering the aisles like a hermit in the desert, so thirsty you'd drink sand if it was put in front of you.

Start smart. First of all, many grocery stores are so vast that they have two entrances. Locate the one that drops you at the produce section. This should always be the first stop. Load up that cart with a lot of colorful fruits and veggies. It's basically the only part of the store your BFB should roam freely. To make sure he doesn't wander off while you pick out your fave five, encourage him to select a fruit he's never tried before, such as star fruit or pomegranate. Experiencing new things as a couple is fun!

Go organic. Next, hit up the organic or natural section of the store. There are lots of great high-fiber pastas and slimming snacks, so browse this aisle before filling the wagon with less-healthy options. Here you'll find things such as BBQ-flavored soy chips—yummy alternatives to greasy potato chips—and freeze-dried fruits (which, with a little cajoling, might eventually replace his candy).

Deli detour. Go ahead and take a number. The lean, low-sodium turkey breast or low-fat cheeses are worth the wait. They taste just as good and will help cut down on some of that sodium and calories deli meats are notorious for. Also, ask for everything thinly sliced, especially the cheese. This will help shave off calories when you're making a sandwich at home.

Go grain. If you fear the bread aisle, relax. The anti-carb craze has bakers on their toes. There are tons of healthful, high-quality loaves. Look for breads with no fewer than 3 grams of fiber per slice—you can even find his white bread in a low-carb, higher-fiber version!

Center showdown. Once you hit the center of the store, it's time to be on guard. The candy, crackers, and cookies and the chips and soda aisles are pretty much a land mine. Go through them as quickly as possible. The longer you let him ponder and browse, the more fatty foods you'll end up with.

Cold is cool. The frozen foods section has its pluses and minuses. There are lots of great frozen veggies and fruits that don't spoil, many low-fat cheese-covered options that are perfect for an anti-veggie BFB, and the frozen blueberries and strawberries are amazing for smoothies. Just beware of the frozen junk foods, like high-fat mozzarella sticks, carb-loaded TV dinners, and full-fat ice creams.

Dairy delight. You'll find lots of great picks in the dairy case. Stock up on yogurts (FAGE® 0% is amazingly good and has 13 grams of protein per cup), low-fat milk, cottage cheese, and eggs. Check here for whole grain tortillas. They're awesome for making breakfast burritos and quesadillas.

SHOP ONLINE, DROP POUNDS

If the resolve to stick to healthy staples dissolves the second you walk through the supermarket doors, give the store the slip. Research shows that buying groceries with a click of the mouse and having them delivered to your house reduces the total amount of foods in the home, especially the availability of high-fat foods.

Think about it: how often do you pick up a bag of this or box of that, just because you saw it? You end up with items that you had no intention of purchasing before you arrived. And, of course, the less food you have around to mindlessly munch, the better off you'll be.

Shopping online means no more long lines, an extra hour or two to do something you really want, and a smaller pant size. Amazingly awesome, huh? Acme, Albertsons, Stop & Shop, Genuardi's, Giant, and Vons, among others, all offer this slimming service.

LABEL LIBEL

Thought those 30 spritzes of calorie-free butter spray were too good to be true? Well, you were right. Just like a lawyer will spin you 'round with confusing jargon, so too will the food industry. Here's what the FDA says these calorie claims really mean.

CALORIE CLARIFICATION

Calorie-free	Fewer than five calories per serving (but if you have 10 servings, it's closer to 50 than to zero!)
Low calorie	Fewer than 40 calories per serving
Light	50 percent less fat or ⅓ fewer calories

FAT FACTS

Fat-free	Less than ½ gram of fat per serving
Reduced fat	At least 25 percent less fat per serving
Low fat	No more than 3 grams of fat per serving

SUGAR PSYCH-OUT

Sugar-free	Less than ½ gram of sugar per serving
Reduced sugar	At least 25 percent less sugar

SALT SHAKEDOWN

Sodium- or salt-free	Fewer than 5 milligrams per serving
Low sodium	140 milligrams or fewer per serving

CHOLESTEROL CLEAR UP

Cholesterol free	No more than 2 milligrams of cholesterol and 2 grams or less of saturated fat
Reduced cholesterol	At least 25 percent less cholesterol and 2 grams or less of saturated fat

MEAT MEANINGS

Lean	Fewer than 10 grams of fat per serving
Extra lean	Fewer than 5 grams of fat per serving

Note: *Free* can also be seen as *zero*, *no*, or *without*. *Low* can also mean *little*, *few*, or *low source of*. *Reduced* can also mean *less*, *lower*, or *modified*.

CHECK BEFORE BUYING

When shopping, check packages for the following artificial sweeteners—ahem, chemicals!—hidden in foods. If you see them, think twice before buying, since they can cause weight gain (see chapter 3 for a refresher!). The most common artificial sweeteners include acesulfame K, aspartame (brand names: NutraSweet and Equal), saccharin (brand name: Sweet 'N Low) and sucralose (brand name: Splenda).

Yes, it's hard to avoid artificial sweeteners at first, especially if you've been stockpiling your cart with "sugar-free" foods and guzzling diet soda. But think of it this way: It's not just about calories at the end of the day. A little sugar isn't going to kill you. Stick to natural sweeteners and smaller servings—your body deserves the real thing!

Here are a few easy changes: Instead of reaching for "light" yogurts, buy the all-natural plain versions. Add a dollop of jam, real fruit, or a few spoonfuls of a sugar-sweetened yogurt. Instead of diet soda, try bubbly seltzer water—just make sure you don't grab the artificially sweetened waters!—with a twist of lemon or lime or a splash of juice.

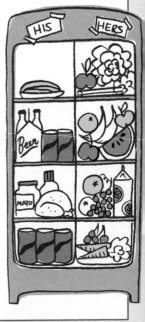

MAKE A DEAL

Relationships are all about compromise—and that goes for grocery shopping, too. So if he wants to throw junk in the cart, try the following replacements instead. No, they're not all fruits and veggies (if you can get him to swap out a mocha-fudge brownie for a bunch of bananas, your powers of reasoning and mind control go way beyond the confines of these pages) but this is real-life we're talking here. And when it comes to BFBs, every little bit helps.

HE WANTS	Chips
Buy	Soy chips (they still have all the good flavors: BBQ, ranch, cheddar cheese)
Why	They've got calcium and protein but aren't full of grease.

HE WANTS	Macaroni and cheese
Buy	Whole wheat or natural brands
Why	You can still satisfy his macaroni and cheese craving while sneaking in some wholesome grains and fiber.

HE WANTS	Eggo Buttermilk waffles
Buy	Kashi GoLean Original waffles
Why	They have six times the fiber, half the fat, and three more grams of protein than the kiddie version.

HE WANTS	Kellogg's Frosted Flakes
Buy	Kellogg's Frosted Flakes Gold Energy
Why	This painless swap has two extra grams of fiber and 1 gram less of sugar.

HE WANTS	Peanuts
Buy	Peanuts in the shell
Why	You'll both eat less when you have to de-shell the nut instead of just grabbing a handful and shoveling them in.

HE WANTS	Brownies
Buy	Warm Delights Mini Molten Chocolate Cake
Why	It's only 150 calories per serving, so even if you decide you want one, it will have hundreds of calories fewer than the half pan of brownies you probably would've consumed (not to mention the licks of batter before popping it in the oven).

HE WANTS	M&M's
Buy	Dark chocolate M&M's
Why	Dark chocolate—not white or milk chocolate—is full of potent antioxidants, and studies have shown it can even lower blood pressure.

HE WANTS	A pint of Ben & Jerry's Cookie Dough ice cream
Buy	Ben & Jerry's single-serving of Cookie Dough ice cream
Why	The feeds-four pint freezes over your diet at a hefty 1,080 calories and 60 grams of fat! The single-serving size is a much safer treat at 240 calories and 13 grams of fat. Especially if you share!

HE WANTS	Cheetos
Buy	Baked! Cheetos Crunchy Cheese Flavored Snacks
Why	Since they're baked, not fried, you save 30 calories and 5 grams of fat per serving.

HE WANTS	Chips Ahoy! Chocolate Chip cookies
Buy	Chips Ahoy! Thin Crisps 100-calorie packs
Why	Obviously, portion control. A single serving of the regular cookies—and who eats just one serving?—is 160 calories.

BFB FINAL THOUGHT
....

Sometimes it's okay to tell a little lie. . . if it will keep you both a little healthier.

We're putting everything up on the conveyor belt. Reaching for the apples, I notice a bag of Double Stuf Oreos for the first time. I pick up the crinkly package, about to ask my honey how these high-fructose corn syrup, artificially-flavored cookies made their way into our cart. The last time they ended up in my cupboard, I ate half a sleeve that very night, standing at the counter with a glass of milk and the knowledge that I had crossed the line from merely snacking occasionally on his treats to leaving him with mere crumbs.

"You know what?" I try to say casually, hoping he'll bite. "I heard these are made with lard." Lard is one word he relates to, thanks to the lovely and super-visual term "lard-ass."

My BFB looks up from the magazine he's reading. "Lard? Really?"

Sometimes it works in my favor that he's too unmoti-vated to bother turning over the package. But his face is so innocent and interested that I feel a twinge of guilt. Well, I reason with myself, after I consume 12 of them, they might as well be made of lard.

"Yeah, the white stuff. It's like sugar and lard in the middle. You're licking sugar-flavored lard."

"Why do you gotta tell me this stuff?" He takes the package from me and sits it on top of the candy display. "What reason will I have to drink milk?"

"Well, you don't wanna eat lard, do you?"

He kisses me on the cheek. "No. I guess I don't. Wouldn't want you to either . . . somehow, I remember you eating quite a few of these last time."

I cough and busy myself with emptying the last few things. He loads the bagged goods into the cart, his mind already turning toward what we're making for dinner, his Double Stufs forgotten. Now, if I can only convince him that there's blubber in the Ben & Jerry's.

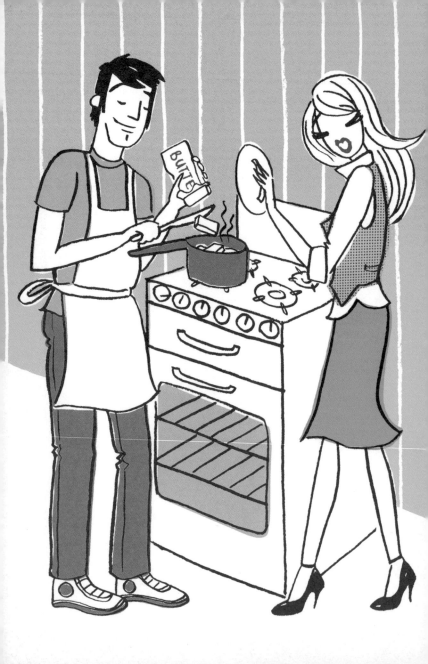

CHAPTER 7

KITCHEN WARS

He's standing over the stove, his curly head bent in concentration, wrinkles across his forehead. "Hand me another piece of cheese?"

"Another one?" He's already put two slices into the pot.

"Yeah, just one more."

I look over my shoulder. The cheese is, seriously, three inches away from him. But he is so focused on stirring that he doesn't even notice. One would think he was making a French delicacy, a soufflé or some other dish worthy of a sous-chef. But, no. My BFB is making— *creating*, as he'd like to think of it—his specialty: SpagettiO gumbo.

Right. So, SpagettiOs. But with things mixed in.

This pride-inducing dish includes the mushy, pasta-in-a-can with tin-flavored sauce that he's been consuming since age four, "culinary" spices (salt and pepper), maybe some cooked chicken if I happen to have some—he never has much besides condiments in his fridge—and, the most necessary, the most dire, the one ingredient without which the gumbo cannot exist: cheese. This dairy product seems to be the one ingredient that constitutes cooking. If he melts it, he has, indeed, cooked.

Of course, he doesn't just make some weird version of SpagettiOs. Oh, no. My BFB is multitalented. If he's manning the stove, I also have a chance of eating an egg sandwich—also smothered in cheese—or, if the night is incredibly special and he's looking to impress—a chicken quesadilla, devoid of anything other than chicken and cheese.

Here's the problem: I am in a constant battle to reduce calories, and he is continually fighting to add more—of everything. His rationale is an innate male belief that more cheese, more butter, more . . . whatever will only make everything taste better.

A BFB doesn't understand—or, sometimes even more alarmingly, care—how many calories he adds to an egg if he plops a blob of butter on the pan to grease it. He doesn't realize that putting three pieces of cheese on an egg sandwich is making it more than just "melty"—it's making it 300 calories closer to the caloric equivalent of a Big Mac. When he's cooking, calories don't even enter his mind.

High-calorie cooking is dangerous to your heart and hips. Homemade meals should be the most delicious, nutrient-packed, and low-cal food you and your man eat. But that doesn't mean you have to be Betty Crocker and he has to be Emeril. There's no need to start from scratch or grow the veggies in the backyard to make something tasty and super healthy.

It's all about simple, nutrient-packed—and delicious!— ingredients. Things that don't go bad in a week, won't take hours to clean up, and won't be able to be resisted once he smells them cooking. Here's everything you need to know to get in and out of the kitchen fast—while still fueling your body with awesome, good for (both of) you food.

YOUR WEAPONS

There are lots of tricks to shorten the time spent preparing, cooking, and cleaning up. The less hassle it takes, the more likely you'll be to actually use the food you bought at the store instead of calling for delivery. Here's what every pseudo-chef should have in his or her arsenal.

Nine-inch and 12-inch nonstick pans. The 9-inch pan is perfect for cooking eggs or sautéing a single chicken breast. A 12-inch pan is great for stir-fries and when you're cooking for both of you. Make sure to invest in these; the better the pan, the less butter, oil, or nonstick spray you'll need, and the less time you'll spend at the sink afterward!

Grill. Whether it's the real thing or a little indoor one (like a George Foreman), a grill is a must for BFBs. It's the one thing he loves to do that's actually good for him, so encouraging its use is a good idea!

Blender. Whip up yummy, low-fat, high-protein smoothies, and low-fat salad dressings, and liquidate fruits and veggies with ease. A blender is a must for the covert cook!

Cooking bags. Steaming rocks. It's totally easy (chicken and veggies steam in minutes), there are no dishes to wash, and it doesn't entail any added fat or calories.

Pizza pan. It's a favorite of BFBs, and, with hardly any work, you can whip up a healthy pie for you and your guy.

FREEZER FRONT LINE

The freezer should be your new best friend. Busy schedules don't leave time for lots of trips to the grocery store, and there's nothing worse than buying enough fruits and veggies to fill a farmer's stand only to see them spoil before you have a chance to eat them—something that's easy to do when the daunting task of cleaning, chopping, and cooking discourages you from actually preparing them. So make sure to have these three essentials frozen at all times:

Proteins. Keep at least one pack of chicken breasts and one pack of ground beef on standby. If you have enough foresight to know that you'll want to cook it when you get home from work, transfer it from the freezer to the fridge in the morning so it's ready to go when you get home. If you don't realize it until you walk through the door, plop the unopened package in a bowl of warm water to speed up the thawing process, or pop it in the microwave to defrost.

Veggies. Diced onions and diced green peppers make an awesome snack on nights when you don't have—or can't stand the thought of cutting and cleaning up— fresh ones. They add a punch of flavor to stir-fries, omelets, Italian dishes, burgers, and just about anything else. Green beans, sugar snap peas, broccoli, and cauliflower are all great to keep on hand for fast and healthy side dishes.

Fruit. Frozen strawberries and blueberries are naturally sweet and perfect for quick smoothies or as bases in desserts. They can also be blended and folded into pancakes and waffles for a delicious, healthy breakfast.

SNEAK ATTACK!

You love him, and you want his heart to beat for years to come. Unfortunately, watching him eat makes your own heart hurt. If you've done everything you can to cajole him into eating good-for-him foods, you're not alone. Stop suggesting, nagging, and giving him looks: do both of you a favor and start sneaking little shots of nutrition into his dishes.

Veggie wars. There are so many wonderful vegetables, from asparagus to squash to zucchini. And here's the best part: though tasty and delicious on their own accord, they are bland enough to be easily camouflaged (with a little trick or two) in many of his go-to dishes.

Making burgers? Mix in a half cup of low-sodium V8 or, believe it or not, baby food—you'll never find a more blended version of carrots, sweet potatoes, or any other good-for-him veggie. (Of course, if you have the time and feel like channeling Martha Stewart—and he's not within earshot!—you can blend the hell of out of cooked tomatoes, carrots, cauliflower, or whichever veggies you can get your hands on.) Another way to get veggies into that meat: toss in some finely diced green peppers and onions (super-easy if you thaw the frozen ones!) and he's just had another serving of veggies he'll never know about! Note: If he's a consistency freak, skip the peppers and onions and just go with the veggie juice or pureed veggies.

Tossing together spaghetti? Grab that V8 and add a cupful to the sauce. Let it simmer, stirring until you are happy with the consistency. If he won't balk at any sort of "lumps," add canned tomatoes and a few sautéed peppers and onions. This trick works well in every red-sauce dish (such as lasagna, chili, and even soups), and you can use carrot juice or other less-vibrant veggies in breads and muffins. If you're using store-bought V8, make sure it's the low-sodium version, or you'll wipe out the veggie benefits with salt!

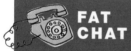

FAT CHAT

TIPS—AND COMPLAINTS!—ON COOKING FROM REAL WOMEN LIKE YOU

"He's a great cook, but his food is usually heavy in the fatty-meat department. So I try to cook healthy foods, and he's a good sport about trying them. The only problem is that an hour after one of my healthy veggie meals, he's in the kitchen munching on some beef jerky or making a mammoth milkshake!" —Emily, 25

"I try to cook healthy and if he's hungry enough, he'll at least try it! Sometimes he just makes faces—veggie burgers especially—but occasionally I'll make something healthy he likes. I've also learned to hide food packages so he won't know if something is supposed to be 'healthy' or not!" —Jill, 28

"Make him a romantic, healthy dinner. If you cook for him and play it up to be a 'date night,' he will feel too bad to pick at the veggies and order a pizza!" —Emily, 25

Fortify with fruit. It's sweet, it usually needs nothing more than a rinse before eating, and yet, getting him to eat three a day is as hard as getting him to put the seat down. But fruit can be worked into just about any bread. Pancakes, waffles, cookies, cake, brownies—all can be used to carry healthy nutrients into his belly. Mash any combo of blueberries, strawberries, raspberries—again, frozen types are best to keep around, since they won't spoil—or bananas. If the recipe calls for one cup of oil, replace half with fruit!

Pump up protein. If you cringe every time he shovels down carb-heavy stacks of pancakes, break out those tricks for waist-friendly weekend breakfasts. Pancakes, waffles, and other bread products have lots of room for protein. Add a half scoop of vanilla-flavored whey protein, a half cup of high protein yogurt (such as FAGE® 0%), or cottage cheese to give substance to those carb-loaded breakfasts. The extra protein will help keep his midafternoon stomach growls at bay.

Increase the fiber. The more fiber in meals, the better. You'll feel fuller longer and, most likely, consume fewer calories. Sprinkle a few tablespoons of ground flaxseed into everything from pizza dough and pancakes to smoothies. Or sprinkle a fiber supplement like Benefiber—it's tasteless and odorless—into just about anything, from sauces and soups to cookies and cappuccino.

CONQUER THE CARBS

Carbs, carbs, carbs. You love 'em but hate what they do to your backside. At this point, pretty much everyone knows eating too many carbs leads to too many extra pounds. But honestly, some carbs get a bad rap. They can be healthy and full of nutrients. The problem arises when you consume *refined* carbs—see chapter 3 for more info on why those should be avoided—and make them the main meal instead of second fiddle to lean protein and, best of all, veggies. So here are some easy, healthier/low-carb alternatives for some of his—and your—favorite foods.

. . . .

Instead of: Spaghetti

Try: House Foods Tofu Shirataki Noodles (Find them at Whole Foods, Trader Joe's, and Asian markets)

Why: There are only 40 calories in the entire 8-ounce pack and 6 carbs, 4 of which are fiber!

Even better: Spaghetti squash. Just cut it in half and bake upsidedown on a cookie sheet at 350°F for 45 minutes or until insides are tender. Score with a fork and presto! Veggie pasta!

Why: The juice of this awesome veggie contains extracts that may help reduce symptoms of an enlarged prostate, which can cause problems in the bathroom and the bedroom. So, if he wants to keep his sexual prowess powerful, encourage him to try it.

Instead of: Lasagna noodles

Try: Whole-wheat or multigrain varieties

Why: There's almost three times the fiber in whole-wheat pasta than regular types.

Even better: Zucchini. Cut lengthwise and layer in pan where noodles would have been.

Why: It's super low in calories and full of fiber, which may help prevent colon cancer.

. . . .

Instead of: A hamburger bun or hotdog roll

Try: A high-fiber tortilla

Why: The flat, less-dense, high-fiber wrap will cut down on some of the carbs hiding in those UFO-sized, super-puffy buns.

Even better: Wrap the burger in lettuce or hand him a fork and a knife and enjoy the meat sans flour.

Why: Even fewer carbs! So if he really wants that starchy side of a potato, it's like breaking even.

. . . .

Instead of: Potatoes

Try: Yams (or sweet potatoes)

Why: These orange-colored beauties are an excellent source of vitamin C and beta-carotene, two powerful antioxidants that help eliminate cell-damaging free radicals that can lead to colon cancer and heart disease.

Even better: If you're making mashed, forget the potatoes all together. Shake a bag of frozen cauliflower into a bowl and pop it in the microwave until soft. Swirl it in a blender with milk, a bit of butter and whichever spices you feel like—garlic, salt, and pepper—and boom: mashed "potatoes."

Why: You're saving tons of carbs and getting all the benefits of this cancer-preventing power veggie.

. . . .

Instead of: White rice

Try: Brown rice

Why: White rice starts out as brown rice—until it's stripped of almost all of its B vitamins, half its manganese and phosphorous, and all its fiber and essential fatty acids—all nutrients that help the body create energy, prevent cancer, and promote a healthy weight. What's left has the nutritional value of cardboard. Not to mention that white rice is a refined carb and spikes blood sugar and insulin levels.

Even better: Cauliflower. Just like potatoes, cauliflower can masquerade as this carb. Either cut very finely with a knife—you'll need a fresh, raw head to start with this time—or use a food processor to shred into the size of rice granules. Steam or toss in the microwave (no need to add water) on high until soft.

Why: Again, you'll cut carbs and get cancer-fighting nutrients.

. . . .

Instead of: Bleached, all-purpose flour

Try: Whole-wheat flour

Why: It has more nutrients and fiber than the super-refined all-purpose flour, because it's derived from the complete wheat kernel, which holds the bran and germ. Try halving the amount of all-purpose flour in cookies, breads, pancakes, waffles, and muffins and make up the difference with whole wheat. It will make foods a little denser and add a yummy nutty flavor.

Even better: Toss in some oats, too. You can grind them in the blender to make oat flour or buy it at a local health-food store.

Why: Studies show that oats lower blood cholesterol and stabilize blood sugar. They're also an awesome replacement for breadcrumbs in dishes like meatloaf!

PANTRY STRATEGY

Here's what you should have on hand at all times. Not only will these ingredients add tons of flavor the easiest possible way—no cutting, chopping, or cleaning!—they also provide amazing health benefits. Here's a list of what to grab at the store and toss in a closet, the fridge, or the freezer until you suddenly want to whip up something that will have that boy's mouth watering without him ever knowing how fabulous it is for him!

Balsamic vinegar: Vinegar has been found to help the body respond more efficiently to insulin. Use it for a tangy flavor on strawberries, seafood, salads, and veggies.

Black peppercorn: As bad as salt can be for you, black pepper is good! It shocks taste buds into sending a message to the stomach that it's time to eat, which causes more hydrochloric acid secretion. This helps with digetion and also decreases gas. (A great thing for BFBs!)

Celery seed: Don't feel like washing and cutting a stalk? Sprinkle this in tuna fish salad and soups. It acts as a natural diuretic and has vitamin C, which helps boost the immune system.

Cinnamon: Spice up pancakes, waffles, French toast, muffins, breads, rice pudding, or oatmeal or add a dash to coffee. Cinnamon helps prevent blood clots and stimulates cells to respond to insulin more efficiently, which aids in the prevention of type 2 diabetes by stabilizing blood sugar.

Dried chili pepper: This powerful pepper may lower the risk of type 2 diabetes, boost immunity, increase metabolism, prevent stomach ulcers, and inhibit the spread of prostate cancer. Sprinkle chili peppers into foods — chili, pizza, quesadillas, and other dishes — that could use a little heat.

107

bfb real-life story

This savvy sweetheart keeps things healthy in the kitchen by whipping up low-fat Mediterranean meals— and keeping her BFB away from the stove!

"If he did the cooking, we'd probably *lose* weight," says Liz, 29, who recently tied the knot with her BFB. "Ninety percent of what he makes is inedible. When he lived on his own, he didn't buy regular pasta—he bought mac and cheese and didn't use the chemical cheese powder. On any given day he had about 20 packets of the junk just lying around!" Liz now tries to keep things healthy by cooking mostly Mediterranean meals. "I really like cooking. Lately, I've been doing a lot of sautéing in olive oil and garlic," she says, happy that Jason is open to trying new things after seeing his own parents experience health problems from years of unhealthy eating. "He tends to dump Old Bay on vegetables—which I'm trying to curtail because of the sodium—so I'm trying to find ways to make my steamed veggies tastier!"

Dried orange peel: Add a bit of orange zest to fruit smoothies, muffins, and even chicken dishes to reap big benefits. The peel is 20 times more powerful than the fruit's juice, and research shows it may lower cholesterol, too.

Ground flaxseed: This increasingly popular seed is full of Omega-3 fatty acids, which may reduce symptoms of everything from asthma to migraines. Flaxseed strengthens bones, is full of fiber, and protects against diabetes, cancer, and heart disease. Add it to muffins, cookies, pizza dough, and hot or cold cereals.

Lemon or lime juice: High in vitamin C, both juices boost the immune system, and lime juice has been shown to have antibiotic effects. Grab a few bottles of lemon or lime juice and toss 'em in the fridge. Both enhance the flavors of other foods, such as chicken and veggies, without adding an ounce of fat. Squirt them on stir-fries in place of oil and use in marinades and salad dressings.

Minced garlic and garlic powder: Garlic has been found to lower blood pressure, fight heart disease, and ward off colds by boosting the immune system. Use it in pasta sauces, burgers, and stir-fries.

Minced onions: Onion is a great starter for so many dishes. It's also a good source of the trace mineral chromium, which may help cells respond to insulin and lower blood sugar. Brown minced onions in a pan before pouring in eggs to kick up an omelet, toss them with a mix of veggies for a stir-fry, or add them with some green peppers to meatloaf.

Oregano: This spice has so many benefits that some health stores actually sell oregano oil. Not only does it fight bacteria, but it also has been shown to have 42 times more antioxidant power than apples and 12 times more than oranges! So sprinkle it on pizza, Italian dishes like spaghetti and lasagna, and in olive oil–based salad dressings.

Paprika: This bright red spice may lower blood pressure, and it contains antioxidants that fight cell damage. Use it to add color to chicken dishes, chili, barbecue, and Mexican dishes.

Pure vanilla extract: Heating up things in the kitchen may heat up the bedroom, too! Not only has vanilla's aroma been found to reduce stress, it's also considered to be an aphrodisiac. Sweeten up smoothies, muffins, cakes, and breads sans sugar by adding a drop or two to the batter.

FAST FIXES

Cut fat and calories in any dish with these little trimming tweaks. The best part? He'll never notice!

Applesauce and other fruit purées: Use applesauce in place of butter or oil in cookies and muffins.

Boiling water: Before adding crumbled hamburger meat to any sauce, toss it in a strainer and pour boiling water over it to cut fat.

Canadian bacon: Canadian bacon has one-third less fat than regular bacon because it's cut from the loin, the leanest part of the pig. Use it in breakfast sandwiches, BLTs, and any recipe that calls for bacon.

Egg whites: Cut cholesterol in omelets, egg sandwiches, and any baked good by using two egg whites for every egg.

Evaporated skim milk: Use it in place of cream in recipes and even tea or coffee. It's fat-free but still thick and creamy!

Fat-free chicken broth: Instead of adding fat to mashed potatoes or stuffing, keep things flavorful and moist with canned chicken broth.

High-heat canola cooking spray: Use this spray in place of margarine or oil to cut tons of calories in everything from eggs to stir-fries.

BE SMART ABOUT SWEETS

Stop reaching for sugar or one of those colored packets. There are two natural alternatives you can use in the kitchen that are even better for you: stevia and agave nectar.

Stevia is a zero-calorie sweetener derived from an herb native to Paraguay. Until recently, it was only available in the vitamin and supplement aisle of health-food stores. But you'll now find a form of stevia sold under the brand-name Truvia in most stores. Use in it in anything from coffee to yogurt to baked goods.

Agave nectar—also called agave syrup—is another all-natural alternative. It does have calories, but it has a lower glycemic index than sugar. (This means it doesn't cause such a rapid spike in blood sugar and can help keep pounds at bay.) Drizzle over yogurt, sweeten iced tea, or swap out maple syrup and use for pancakes.

FAT FLASH

Olive oil is known for its health benefits, but not all bottles are created equal. Be sure to buy extra virgin or virgin, for these are the least processed forms and are best at removing cancer-causing agents from the body. Just remember, "light" doesn't mean lower in calories. It just has a lighter color and flavor.

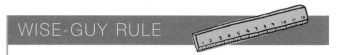

WISE-GUY RULE

Make him love you forever and cook with his all-time favorite ingredient: beer. An enzyme in hops has cancer-fighting properties, so even though he thinks he's getting a treat—and not complaining so much about the veggies—you know you're both eating something pretty damn good for you, too.

BFB FINAL THOUGHT

As long as he's eating something healthy, it doesn't really matter how he eats it.

"Do you like it?" I pull the spoon away from his mouth, hoping the little pre-dinner taste-test will prove positive. He thumbs away a bit of sauce from his lower lip, nodding as he thinks about it.

"Yeah," he says, "It's good."

I cock my head to the side. "Seriously? You don't like it?"

It had been quite a few weekends since I'd cooked anything, and I had felt like experimenting with a tomato sauce (seasoned with onion, basil, and garlic, all from the spice cabinet!). I planned to add chunks of chicken and serve it over tofu noodles. I was thrilled he finally agreed to try something with the word *tofu* in it. But getting him to like it was going to be another story.

As I fix our plates, he asks me cautiously "Can I just have the chicken and sauce on the side, on a separate plate?"

"You don't want it on the noodles?" I ask.

"No. I'll just put ketchup on those."

I look at him, always amazed at his strangeness. This is a human being who prefers to slobber down spaghetti with a slick sheen of ketchup rather than risk a marinara that might have the tiniest sliver of actual tomato.

I sigh. "Okay . . ."

I slide our plates onto the table and watch as he happily squirts ketchup onto his noodles. He slurps down the first bite and then looks up, surprised.

"Hey, this is pretty good."

I laugh, happy he likes it.

"You should really try it with ketchup," he insists. "So good."

I shake my head, sip my wine, and wonder if our kids will be as screwed up as he is.

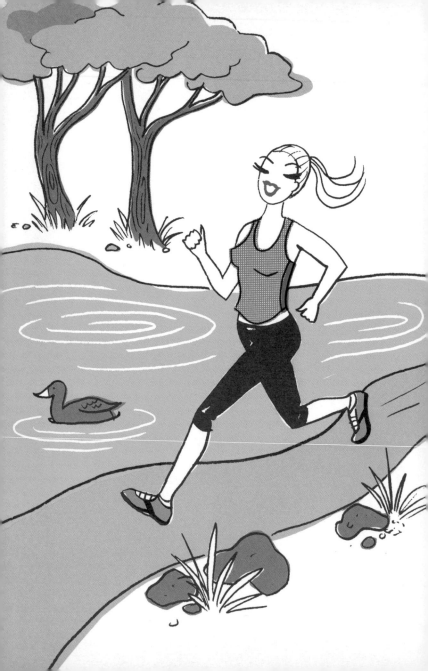

CHAPTER 8

YOU GOTTA MOVE IT, SISTER

Exercise. Most likely, you love it or hate it. If you're from the I-hate-to-miss-a-workout camp, keep it up. If, however, you can think of a billion other things you'd rather do than break a sweat, we need to talk. No, not in the "you're in trouble" sort of way, but honestly: You're missing out. Big time.

Believe it or not, humans weren't designed to sit in cubicles and click away at e-mail for eight hours a day. The body is a machine and it actually *wants* to move. Working out can be fun, feel amazing, and double as a stand-in for your body's protector, therapist, and life coach, all rolled into one.

If you've never experienced the fun side of working out, don't roll your eyes and flip to the next chapter. This section is here to change all that—and to keep you motivated and teach you ways to get an even better workout if you're already a devotee! Because no matter how you feel about working out, the hard truth is this: You can't get something for nothing. If you want to stay healthy and enjoy your body, you're going to have to get off the couch (or that desk chair!) a little bit every day. Here's why you should be moving, how to get the most out of your time, and how to have fun doing it!

WHY YOU GOTTA MOVE

Everyone knows that working out will help you look good in a bathing suit and slip into those skinny jeans whenever you please. But there are so many more reasons to break a sweat than to simply rock a rockin' bod. (Not that there's anything wrong with that being the biggest motivator!) Check out all these awesome extras you get in addition to a hottie's body.

Increased energy. With work, friends, family, quality BFB time, and, let's be honest, just keeping yourself fed and in clean clothes, life can feel like a nonstop marathon. It can be more than a little hard to push yourself to work out. But the more you move, the more energy you'll have. Research shows that regular exercise boosts energy levels and decreases fatigue. So stop subsisting on caffeine and log a few miles instead.

The power to shape-shift. Whatever exercise you choose—Pilates, hiking, yoga, surfing, Spinning, dancing, skiing, kick boxing, rollerblading, weights, running—if you commit to regular workouts, you have the power to change the shape and look of your body by elongating those muscles, toning those triceps, and whittling that waist.

A bigger smile. Research shows that logging regular sweat sessions lessens feelings of depression. Each time you work out, endorphins (hormones found in the brain that cause happy, positive feelings) increase. So if you're down, frustrated, or just ready to kill your BFB, head to the gym.

A calorie-burning bod. The more lean muscle mass on your body, the more calories you'll burn—doing nothing! That's because it takes energy (i.e., calories) to maintain those rock-hard abs. Studies estimate that a pound of muscle burns up to 50 calories per day. So if you add on three pounds of muscle, that's 150 extra calories per day that you'll torch while watching way too much reality TV.

More chances to do whatever you want. Think of each minute on the treadmill as an investment in years to come. Heart disease is the number one killer of women in the United States. Working out fights the risk of heart disease and lessens your chance of developing type 2 diabetes and other obesity-related health issues.

Strong bones. Don't end up with a broken hip by the time you're 50. Weight-bearing exercises, including walking, jogging, running, dancing, and weight-lifting, keep bones strong.

Increased endurance. Forget heading home from the mall early or catching your breath at the top of the stairs! The more you work out, the more conditioned your heart becomes, which gives you the ability to do other things longer and better.

Float above the stress. Rough day at work or a fight with your BFB? Hit the gym. You'll reduce the amount of stress hormones coarsing through your body, resulting in relaxed blood vessels, lower blood pressure, and a slower heart rate. Exercise also increases the amount of serotonin in the brain, a chemical that helps keep you calm.

Gorgeous skin. Those 90 minutes on your yoga mat or your daily treadmill training session improves circulation and increases oxygen to your skin, which helps boost the production of collagen, the connective tissue that keeps skin looking youthful. Sweating also releases toxins—nasty things like cigarette smoke and air pollution—and unclogs pores, which means clearer, healthier skin.

Become unstoppable. Making it through an entire spin class or hiking to the top of a mountain shows you can accomplish anything you set your mind to—and that goes for outside the gym, too. So get ready to ask for that promotion or leave your job for the one you really want!

More sick days . . . to use for fun! Exercise boosts your immune system, which means catching fewer colds and flus. And when you do get sick, bouncing back faster.

All As. Increased blood flow and oxygen to the brain helps with quick thinking.

Better Zs. If restless nights have you on the verge of becoming addicted to over-the-counter sleep meds, log some gym time. It helps you fall asleep easier and feel more rested when you wake.

A rockin' love life. Not only does exercise increase confidence, which makes you more able to let go of reservations between the sheets and enjoy yourself and your partner, but a study by the University of British Columbia found that women who exercised for 20 minutes had greater sexual response than their sedentary counterparts. And keeping him moving helps prevent things from going, er, soft. Researchers at the Harvard School of Public Health reported that active men had a 30 percent lower chance of erectile dysfunction.

SO, HOW MUCH DO YOU NEED?

It might not be something you want to hear, but to reap the health benefits and ward off those BFB-associated pounds—or lose them!—you should be logging about 200 minutes of heart-pumping activity a week. (It's not as bad as it sounds. That's only 30 minutes a day!) But if you hate the idea of treadmills or gym classes, there are still hundreds of different ways to break a sweat.

Alternate between regular workouts and active "free-bies" that are so fun you don't even realize you're clocking workout time! (Check out the get-fit dates on page 143 for a few ideas.)

MAKE IT A HABIT

Good news: It only takes three weeks to become obsessive-compulsive about something new! (C'mon, everyone's got something, whether it's always getting your morning latte or checking to make sure the coffee pot is off one last time before leaving for work.) So if actually getting your butt to the gym hasn't panned out in the past—as in, you've tried to start an exercise routine more than a few times, only to give it up—it's time to torture yourself for 21 days until it becomes automatic.

It's not as hard as it seems. Try attending a group class. Once you're there, you'll be shocked at how normal it is to be working out—even at 6 A.M.—when there are 20 other people doing it with you. Still afraid you'll miss class? Play up your co-dependent side and ask the instructor to e-mail you the night before (there are some amazing instructors who care enough to do this!). Plan to have a buddy wait for you or, if you can afford it, hire a personal trainer to get you through the first few weeks. If it helps you begin a lifetime of healthy living and lookin' awesome in those jeans, it'll be money well spent.

EARLY-BIRD BOOST

There is nothing better than walking into work, cup of coffee in hand, knowing you've already met your sweat quota for the day—and that there's no treadmill in the way of you and your favorite TV show when you get home! An even bigger reason to roll out of bed early: Research shows that morning exercisers tend to stick with workouts better than those who hit the gym later in the day. That's because the more time that passes between when the alarm blares and when you slip on those sneaks, the more distractions are able to get in the way. A late night at work, a text from the BFB proposing dinner out, a call from a college girlfriend, happy-hour drinks with coworkers—there will always be something to tempt (or flat out demand) you to forfeit your gym time.

Of course, working out at any time is great, as long as you actually do it! If you hate the first light more than a hungover vampire on a Monday morning, you don't have to kick-box at 6 A.M. Just be prepared to do whatever it takes—fib to your boss, pay big bucks for a Pilates class so you won't skip it, pack a bag and go directly from work to the gym—whatever it is that will ensure that you wind up crossing that workout off your list of must-dos before you climb into bed. Because if there's one thing to remember, it's this: Missing one day might not seem like a lot, but all those days you *do* make it to the gym add up to the hot body and healthy heart you want.

WISE-GUY RULE

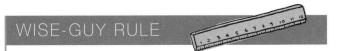

Don't let your BFB derail you. If you're on the way to the gym and the cell rings, don't pick it up if there's even the slightest chance he could sweet-talk you out of Spin class. Instead, text him back something cute, like: "At the gym! Call you back as soon as I'm done!" He'll never know you had no intention of picking up his call. Besides, most men will be more than a little turned on that their lady is keeping herself hot just for him. (At least, that's what they like to think, so we might as well let them!)

SEE RESULTS FASTER

There are three variables at play when it comes to losing that perpetual spare tire: how often you work out, how long you work out, and how hard you work out. In order to get the most out of your exercise, you need to keep your heart beating at or above 70 percent of your maximum heart rate (MHR) for at least 30 minutes. (Your MHR is how fast your heart would be beating in an all-out effort—so, think running at high speeds from a crazy killer in a dark alley or sprinting past massive crowds to grab the last pair of discounted Manolos.) To find your MHR, subtract your age from 226. If you're 25, your MHR would be 201 beats per minute (BPM).

Obviously, how often you break a sweat and how long you stay on the elliptical machine are easy to track. But the only way to truly know you're not slacking off while zoning out on the treadmill is by keeping tabs on your ticker. "Heart-rate monitoring is essential to really reach your fitness goals," says Brooke Hayward, a master Spinning instructor with Mad Dogg Athletics and American Council of Exercise certified aerobics instructor. "Otherwise, it's just a guess if you're accomplishing what you think you are."

Just as you count reps while lifting weights, monitoring your body's most important muscle as carefully will help make the most of your daily workout. There are two ways to check your heart rate:

1 **Buy a heart-rate monitor.** This gotta-get gadget is your new best friend when trying to keep off weight or lose those annoying five pounds that won't seem to budge. It's like having a personal trainer—minus the

crazy price tag and weird spandex outfits—telling you to pick up the pace or ease up a bit.

2 Stay in the zone. If you don't want to spring for a monitor—though if you've been working out religiously and not seeing a difference, it's definitely worth paying $100 for a good one!—check in with yourself throughout your workout by using the workout zones on page 125. They're not as dead-on accurate as a heart-rate monitor, but they will help you push yourself. (However, if you have a friend who owns a monitor, see if you can snag it for a workout or two, just to get an idea of what it feels like to reach 70 percent of your MHR.)

bfb real-life story

After meeting her BFB, this die-hard gym-goer started missing her workouts more and more.

"Our first year together, I stopped working out," admits Jessica, 25, who found herself forfeiting gym time for guy time. "I lived in the city and he lived outside the city, so he would pick me up after work—ridding my schedule of the gym." But, after gaining a few pounds thanks to eating more dinners out and moving less, she realized it was time to get back in gear. "If I'm going to eat like him, I *have* to work out!" Jess and her BFB now live together, so it's easier for her to keep her gym schedule in place—which, happily enough, encourages her man to join her. "He tries harder when I work harder," she says.

YOUR WORKOUT ZONES

Pretty easy: 50 to 60 percent of your MHR. You could easily talk with a friend and not be out of breath. Although you'd have to work out here for big chunks at a time to really burn calories, this zone is still good for improving your overall health.

Starting to sweat: 60 to 70 percent of your MHR. This level is beginning to put some stress on the body, but you could stay at a steady pace for a long period. This zone is great for strengthening the heart and improving endurance.

Killing calories: 70 to 85 percent of your MHR. This is your aerobic or target heart rate zone. It's the fastest pace you can maintain while still being able to say about four words without taking a breath. Stay in this zone for the majority of your workout to burn the most calories without going breathless.

Sprint speed: 85 to 100 percent of your MHR. This is where you body goes anaerobic—it stops using oxygen for energy and the muscles start making lactic acid, which gives you that "Oh my God, my legs are burning!" sensation. You can say only one or two words here without needing to take a breath—you're pretty much gasping when you near your MHR—and can only stay in this zone for a short time without slowing for a recovery. Training in this zone—alternate between one-minute

125

sprints and one minute at a slower pace for 30 to 40 minutes—once or twice a week increases muscle strength and helps keep you ready for quick bursts of speed, in case you actually ever do have to run for something, whether it's the bus or the Manolos!

KNOW YOUR NUMBER

If you have a heart-rate monitor, you'll need to do a little math to find out exactly what your calorie-burning sweet spot is—aka your target heart rate. This is the aerobic range, and 70–85 percent of your MHR. We'll use a fabulous 25-year-old as our example.

1 **First, find your MHR by subtracting your age from 226.** 226 − 25 = 201

2 **Multiply your MHR by 70 percent.** 201 x .70 = 140.7

3 **Multiply your MHR by 85 percent.** 201 x .85 = 170.85

So, to train aerobically, this hottie should keep her heart rate between 140.7 and 170.85 beats per minute for at least 30 minutes. No more counting warm-ups and cool-downs as part of the workout if you really want to banish that belly!

Note: BFBs can find their MHR by subtracting their age from 220 (220 − age = men's MHR).

STAY IN TOUCH

The fitter you become, the more conditioned your heart will be. After three to six months of consistent training, a pace that used to spike that thumper up to, say, 160, will probably get it up to only 145–150 BPM. You'll have to work a little harder to achieve the same level of workout you reached before. And the only way you'll know this for sure is with a heart rate monitor. Without it, you could work out day after day and see no improvement. Even if you buy one, wear it a while, and then forget about it, pull it out every few months to see how you're doing and to avoid stagnating at those terrible plateaus.

DEVELOP YOUR INNER HEALTH VOICE

It's hard enough to stay on track when your BFB is giving you plenty of excuses to skip yoga or step class. But the worst and most devious saboteur is that oh-so-dangerous little voice inside your head. Try these two methods to develop a strong defense.

1 **Play pretend.** Researchers found out years ago that simply cracking a smile can improve your mood. Smile, and you start to feel happy. (Go ahead, try it. Smile. It's a little weird, right? You feel happier!) Telling yourself you *want* to work out works the same way.

You're tired, you're achy, it's been the longest day of your life, and all you want to do is go home, pour a glass of wine, and eat an entire bag of your favorite snack in front of the tube. Instead of giving in, try this mantra: "I'm so excited to go to the gym! I have been waiting all day for this! I LOVE working out." No, you don't have to say it out loud, and it doesn't matter if it's actually the furthest thing from the truth. It's the placebo effect for your bum. By repeating this or any other "I heart the gym" slogan in your head, you'll actually start to feel more up to it!

2 **Ignore yourself.** The alarm goes off. Your first thought is: "I cannot do it. Not today. I need sleep." So, you're tired. Okay, you're *exhausted*. That's fine. Go ahead and let that little mantra play inside your head. But the entire time it's running, quietly get up, walk to your dresser, drag the sports bra over your head, pull on the pants, blindly grab a T-shirt (at this hour, matching is not expected or necessary), and slip on the shoes. By the time you're driving to the gym or walking downstairs to the treadmill, the voice may still be insisting: "You're crazy! Who works out at this time? Nut jobs! That's who!" But soon, it dwindles to something like: "Fine. I'm going, but I'm not doing a lot. I'll just go slow today, you hear me? No sprinting." Even if you do have a less intense day, it's still something. But chances are, once you've been up for 10 or 15 minutes, you'll be fine—and a lot happier that you got your workout in. Especially

when you get stuck in traffic on the way home from work that night and realize you would have ended up missing sweat time!

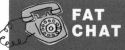

FAT CHAT

WHAT REAL WOMEN LIKE YOU THINK ABOUT THE GYM

"I feel amazing after I work out. When I can't make it to the gym, my eating habits become more and more unhealthy. I think it may be because when I work out, I feel like I would wreck it if I ate a huge meal." —Elena, 21

"I'm always energized after a workout, and when I don't go to the gym, I get angry with myself." —Carly, 21

"He's not motivated to exercise at all, so when I'm in a slump or not motivated, he's not there to push me to go for that jog. I don't work out less; it can just be hard to do it when he's watching TV." —Melissa, 25

"I do yoga twice a week, 40 or more minutes of cardio most other days, and ride my bike everywhere within five miles. I really hate missing a workout. Working out makes me feel less anxious, more focused, and a healthy tired." —Liz, 29

"I feel great after a workout! The days I miss it, I usually feel lousy and am more likely to binge eat." —Joy, 21

"I like working out, but I wouldn't mind getting the same healthy benefits by taking a pill if it were at all possible." —Susan, 52

"I like to make it to the gym at least five days a week. When I miss, it's okay, I just need to compensate by eating a little less food that day." —Jessica, 25

STRIKE A POSE

A study funded by the National Cancer Institute found that overweight people who practiced yoga lost about five pounds during the same time that those not hitting the mat gained 14 pounds. Though science can't fully explain why, many believe it may be because of the amazing mind-body connection that yoga helps you develop over time. As you learn to drop away the non-stop running of your mind and focus only on your breath and body, you learn to be in the moment and take care of your body. Something, experts say, eventually starts to show up in your food choices and helps curb overeating. So say *Om* and tune into what you really need, on—and off—the mat.

BFB FINAL THOUGHT

Remember what you'll be gaining— and losing—if you get your bum to class.

I'm snuggled down under the covers, tucked away from the world. My BFB is beside me, and I've hit that moment when his shoulder feels better than a pillow. I sigh deeply, try to ignore the sunlight, and readjust myself on his shoulder. He opens one eye.

"What time is it?" he mumbles, still mostly asleep.

"Nine."

He frowns. "Go back to sleep. It's Saturday."

"I can't. Yoga."

He holds me tighter. "No. Snuggle time."

I bite my lower lip, tempted. I am *not* feeling yoga right now. Maybe I'll skip just this once . . . .

No. You have to go, my Inner Health Voice insists. *This is the one day of the week you actually have time to make this class. Besides, in 15 minutes he'll be drooling into the pillow and you'll be awake and totally pissed you missed it.*

Dammit. My Inner Health Voice is right. (Thanks, Inner Health Voice.)

Still . . . I have to get past him. He has me by the arms and is threatening tickling. He leaves me with little choice.

"Hey, how about you come with me?" He pauses and I can see his fuzzy brain trying to formulate a good excuse. And then, the "better her than me" reflex that saves BFBs from yoga sessions everywhere kicks in, and his grasp loosens.

I disengage myself from his arms, plant a kiss on his cheek, and hop out of bed. I feel a twinge of guilt for leaving, but I know in two more seconds he'll be snoring. And when we head out to dinner tonight, I'll feel energetic and slim, rather than slothful and pudgy— which will make Saturday night all the more special.

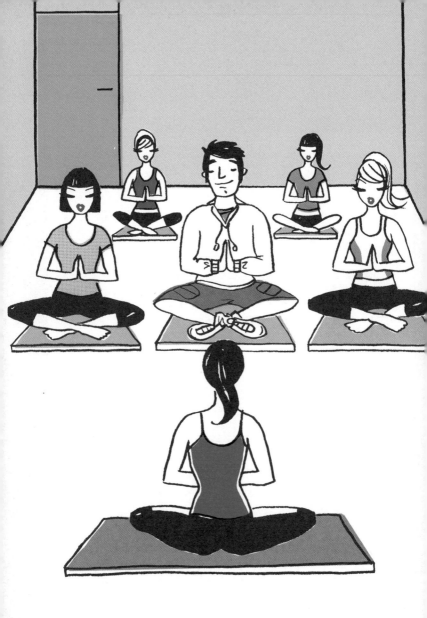

CHAPTER 9

HEALTH-IFY
THAT BOY

"Turn up your gear!" The music's so loud that he can't hear me. He stops pedaling and leans toward me. "What?!"

"Your gear! Turn it up!" I make motions with my hand and then crank up my own gear until my pedals hardly turn. "Like this!"

I have been bugging my BFB to try a Spin class for weeks—*months*—totally sure that if he tried just one, he'd be hooked and we could blissfully attend class together. Now, I'm not sure if it was the best idea. He looks, to put it nicely, like a confused, humongous baby chicken trying out its first few steps. His entire

body is rigid, he's got about zero resistance on the pedals—
which results in a jerky, half-hysterical, half-maddening
break-dance-like cadence—and his face holds the tortured
look of a prisoner of war.

"You owe me pancakes!" he yells as another
Madonna song blares through the speakers. "A lot of
pancakes!" "Okay!" I call back sweetly, even though I'm
cringing internally and thinking that he won't burn off a
single hot cake unless he starts biking with some resistance. I try to ignore him for the rest of class, hoping
he'll stick it out and won't leave midway through.

Somehow, he survives. As we head out, I'm happily
high on endorphins (I think I shut down after the
Madonna song and convinced myself no one knew he
was with me), while he's walking so gingerly you'd think
he was just assaulted in the men's locker room.

"What's wrong?" I finally ask, though I can tell he's
been waiting to tell me since the Material Girl belted her
last chord.

"My balls hurt."

And that was the end of spinning class. It took a few
more not-so-successful attempts to get him to conform to my
workout ways—an embarrassing yoga class (he fell asleep),
jogs that ended in arguments (I wanted to go fast, he wanted
to hold hands), and a totally shut-down DVD workout (he
wouldn't even try it)—before I realized that no matter how

much I cajoled, pleaded, and begged, we just weren't soul mates when it came to gym time. We will never be one of those seemingly perfect couples jogging next to each other in the park. But, in the time that we've been together, my BFB has gone from a total anti-veggie and anti-gym guy to a man who will eat a few bites of salad (baby steps) and will do a good 40 minutes on the treadmill (he actually rigs it so he's holding his video game controller at the same time). But as long as he's doing *something* to get his heart rate up (and he doesn't end up breaking his neck), I'm happy.

Because, let's face it, the healthier your man's habits become, the easier it will be for you to stay slim. Whether he's too friendly with the couch or refuses to eat something other than burgers, fries, and pizza, here's how to help him shape up.

KNOW YOUR GUY

When it comes to getting your BFB healthy, the first thing you gotta know is why he's currently behaving the way he is. There are a few types of guys—some have multiple issues, though we love them anyway, oddly enough. Here's how to deal with each.

The USED-TO-BE-THIN GUY: For the majority of his life, he's been able to eat whatever he wants and still stay thinner than a flagpole. Without an ounce of fat sticking to his ribs, he never felt the need to pay attention to how the junk he was shoveling down might be affecting his insides, like his heart. Then, his twenties hit, he got stuck behind a desk, and his roaring metabolism started to slow. Result: a few too many pounds around his middle.

What he's feeling: Lost and confused. The same burgers and fries he used to devour have turned against him. He's never even thought about ordering a salad or stir-fry when eating out.

What he needs: Nutrition 101. Start explaining—slowly, you don't want to scare him—the basics. Explain why he should increase his daily intake of fruits and veggies (if you start out telling him to cut out his favorite foods, you will most likely be met with resistance). Little by little, introduce him to other aspects. ("Honey, here's the nutritional info, right here on the back of the box. This is how many calories are in a serving. This is how many Cheetos are *actually* a serving.") Little changes can make a huge difference in his health and his belly.

• •

The HAS-ALWAYS-BEEN-THE-BIG-GUY GUY: He's grizzly-bear sized and seems okay with it. But no matter how lovable and comfy his big, burly body may be, the extra weight is doing damage to his heart and putting him at risk for obesity-related issues.

What he's feeling: If the doc hits him with a report of high cholesterol or a prescription to drop a few pounds, he probably feels angry and frustrated. Why can't he be like his friend, what's-his-name, who's never had to deal with a weight issue? Also, he may feel despondent. "I haven't been able to get the weight off before, why will it work now?"

What he needs: Your support. If you live together, start stocking the fridge with healthy alternatives to his favorite foods and making some of his go-to meals a little bit healthier. (See recipes, page 162–167, for ideas.) If you live apart, make suggestions to spend an evening in and cook a healthy dinner together (lots of room for romance!) rather than eating out and overdoing it on appetizers. Also, make dates more active to get him sweating (see page 147 for ideas).

. . . .

The "I'M NOT A MEATHEAD" GUY: He's never stepped foot in the gym and isn't looking to start anytime soon. He hates the idea of working out alongside buff dudes who look like they funnel creatine for breakfast.

What he's feeling: Insecure and inadequate. He's afraid he doesn't measure up to the gym rats and worries he'll look stupid bench-pressing 15 pounds while they're all rocking 150.

137

What he needs: A push to get over his fears. Once he steps foot inside, he'll find out there are a lot more average guys trying to shed pounds than body builders flexing in front of the mirrors. So join a gym together. The buddy system always helps ease I'm-gonna-look-like-a-jerk fears. If he's open to it, schedule a time to meet a personal trainer together (some gyms offer two or three free visits when you join). If his ego is in jeopardy of being hurt, you can shoulder the blame for signing up. If he still refuses to step inside the gym, encourage him to do pickup sports with the guys or start doing a few pushups and crunches every day at home.

. . . .

The ALL-OR-NOTHING GUY: His motto is "Go hard or go home." He starts an exercise program only to overdo it on the first day, injuring his back or another part of himself. Or he cuts out carbs entirely for a week and is so crabby and tired he eventually caves in to a bread binge (which, on top of all that saturated fat he's been consuming, is a killer combo). This knocks him out of commission for the next two weeks, until the cycle starts all over again.

What he's feeling: Frustration and failure. Both are things that can affect his self-esteem.

What he needs: Balance. Remind him that gaining the weight didn't happen overnight and losing it won't either. It's little steps over a long time that will get him where he wants to go. Help him get there by constantly encouraging him to focus on his overall health rather than going to extremes he'll never be able to keep.

. . . .

The "I LOOK GOOD, WHY WORRY?" GUY: This type may be the hardest to convince that his habits need rehab. His body still generates muscles in his sleep, you could bounce a quarter off his abs, and yet to watch him eat makes you cringe. No human being needs that much salt or saturated fat!

What he's feeling: Invincibility. Heart disease, diabetes, and high blood pressure seem like imaginary foes.

What he needs: A seed planted in his head that what he eats now could affect his life later and that you want him to be around as long as possible. Then, try to augment his intake of veggies and low-fat options whenever you can. Cajole him into tasting bites of your favorite dishes and expand his horizons with all the awesome things to eat that aren't fried in grease.

NIX NAGGING

You love him. You want him to be healthy and, let's be honest, you want him to look hot on the beach. But when it comes down to it, there's a line you can't cross if you want to keep your relationship healthy. Start nagging him, and

139

not only will you start to hate that you feel more like a mom than a girlfriend, but he'll start tuning you out or finding ways to appease you without making any real changes.

"I hate putting a napkin on my lap when we go out to eat," says Tom, 21. "But my girlfriend, Kelley, will always get annoyed and bug me to do it. Half the time I put it on the seat next me, just so I can get out of it."

Nobody likes to be told what to do. Instead of resorting to whining, begging, and arguing, try to find a compromise. "My girlfriend has been trying to get me to try Bikram yoga for about a month and a half," says Corey, 26. "But it's 100 degrees in there. I told her being stuck in a small room with sweaty strangers while trying to hold a crane isn't very appealing." But, to make them both happy, they reached a compromise: "We're not going to start with Bikram," says Corey. "She finally understood I have this fear of passing out or vomiting in front of others—it would probably really kill the vibe—so we're going to start with basic yoga instead."

XBOX XS POUNDS

There's still hope for your video-gaming guru. Researchers at the University of Wisconsin have found that playing a few rounds of *Dance Dance Revolution* is just as good as hitting the gym.

The hip-hop dance steps use the large muscle

groups, namely the quads, which work the heart and lungs and kill calories. Play for a half hour and you'll have burned almost 300 calories!

And now, Nintendo has come out with *Wii Fit*, a healthier version of the popular interactive video game. Hop on a balance board—it weighs you and figures out your BMI, too!—and start snowboarding, skiing, boxing, and toning up with yoga. Swap some couch time with playtime a little bit every day and your boy will start to see a difference in his bod. Sure beats Tetris!

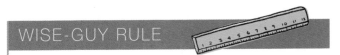

WISE-GUY RULE

Grandma was right: It's what's on the inside that counts. Doctors say that even skinny people can have major deposits of internal fat. No matter how slim he might be, he needs to eat healthy foods and hit the gym a few days a week to prevent hidden obesity, which can lead to heart disease and diabetes.

WHY BRIBES ARE OKAY

If he's dragging his feet to get fit, go ahead and try bribery. A study published in the *Journal of Occupational and Environmental Medicine* reported that overweight employees that were promised financial incentives (read: money!) to drop pounds, lost about two times the weight

141

than those who didn't have a reward coming to them. Although you won't be swiping his palm with green, the promise of tickets to see his favorite band, a night out at his favorite restaurant, or a weekend away where he's always wanted to go, might help him reach his goals.

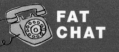

FAT CHAT

TIPS ON HEALTH-IFYNG HIM FROM REAL WOMEN LIKE YOU

"I get silly and kinda jump on him, just to get our energy up. I'm also trying to get him to take me to the zoo. And camping!" — Molly, 21

"He would *never* feel comfortable going to a gym. He doesn't like the thought of people 'staring at him.' So we try and do things like walk around our neighborhood and ride our stationary bike at home." — Melissa, 26

"Snowboarding and skiing are fun dates that burn tons of calories. A full day on the slopes can burn over 1,000 calories!" — Elena, 21

"I've got him eating breakfast — a piece of fruit or yogurt on the go — and drinking water. I'm also proud that I switched him from ground beef to turkey meat and from tacos to taco salads." — Jessica, 25

"Mini golf is always fun — and you're walking, so it gives him some exercise! Bowling will get his arms moving too." — Emily, 26

"I buy a lot of turkey sausage, make a lot of salads and veggies." — Mandy, 28

"He's actually started eating fruit when I leave it out on the counter. You have to lead by example. When I read labels and say 'No, thanks,' to junk, he does too." — Jill, 29

THERE'S MORE THAN DINNER AND A MOVIE

If he hates the idea of "working out," get him moving on the sly. There are lots of fun, active dates the two of you can enjoy. Not to mention that trying something new as a couple helps keep you from hitting a relationship rut. From setting up a Slip 'N Slide to spending the day exploring a new part of the city (on foot!), you'll have an awesome time and work in some activity. Take turns picking the outing — it's only fair that you try camping if he tries ice-skating — and have fun together! Here are some other ideas to get you out of the TV-filled afternoons and big-dinner-out routine.

Be a masseuse. Turn off the TV, light some candles, and give your arms a workout by giving him a back massage he'll never forget. Be careful he doesn't fall asleep — it's your turn next!

Channel TLC. Rearrange the living room or give the kitchen a fresh coat of paint — you'll be doing something creative *and* burning cals! Your guy's not into it? Remind him that studies show that men who do more work around the house are worked over more in bed by their oh-so-appreciative ladies!

Climb a tree. Race each other to the top or, for a more calming day, grab a book and find a branch where you can spend the afternoon reading to each other.

Get a dog. A four-legged friend might be just the inspiration you need to get outside and take a hike or a few laps around the block. Research shows that being responsible for walking a dog can motivate you to become more active, drop extra pounds, increase flexibility, and even boost self-confidence.

Head to a museum. Museums are usually vast buildings with lots of steps (wear comfortable shoes!). You'll learn something new and have lots to talk about. Hello, smart and sexy, goodbye flabby couch-impressioned bum!

Join a team. Softball, kickball, soccer—a local league will give you and your guy a chance to collaboratively win and lose together, not to mention make some like-minded friends. A study published in the *New England Journal of Medicine* found that hanging out with healthy friends can affect your own waistline. If they are active, there's a good chance you will be, too!

Learn to salsa. Or swing or tango or any other form of dance. Not only will you burn calories—up to 10 calories per minute!—but you'll develop a lifetime skill that will give you more options for Saturday nights out. *Olé!*

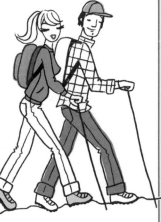

Pound some balls. Spend the evening at the batting cage or driving range. Take turns cheering each other on while you perfect your swing and build strength in your core and arms.

Ride some rides. At the end of the day, your feet will ache from walking back and forth across the parks. Not to mention that those shots of adrenaline you'll get from plummeting will have you both feeling amorous.

See a concert. Singing and dancing to your favorite group will have you feeling good, and, if you stand in the pit, burning major calories. Thirty minutes of moshing will torch about 220 calories!

Stargaze. Grab a few blankets and head outside for the ultimate romantic—and totally cheap!—date. No, you won't be burning off cals, but you'll be away from the TV, and research shows that keeping TV hours to less than 10 a week can keep pounds at bay.

Striptease. All that bending and dancing is such a good workout that gyms across the country have started teaching classes—not to mention this little bit of action will most likely lead to another calorie-burning activity! Just make sure he gives you a show too sometime!

Volunteer. Deliver meals to the homeless, walk the dogs at an animal shelter, or pack boxes at a local food bank—whatever you do, you'll be moving and feeling great for helping others.

Of course, there are a million fun things you and your honey can do together. For more calorie-busting ideas, see the chart on the next page. Just as he can eat more than you, he burns more calories than you when working out, too. So if he tops off a run with a double-scoop cone, you may want to think about staying singular.

BFB FINAL THOUGHT

Don't give up hope—if a garage-band, anti-gym, refuses-to-sweat kid can change for the better, anyone can.

I think I'm in shock. I'm happily running on a treadmill, looking out over New York's Union Square, and three machines down, my BFB is walking at a fast pace, sweat dripping off his forehead. It has taken us three years, 52 days, and a few odd hours, but we have actually joined a gym together. On our key chains now hang one of the most wonderful, unifying little pieces of bright yellow and red plastic I've ever seen: a gym membership card.

He feels me watching him and glances over. I smile and wave. He realizes I'm showing him up, raises an eyebrow, and bumps up his speed, breaking into a little jog. I rise to the challenge, beeping my way up into a faster run. He beeps . . . then I beep . . . we don't stop until we're both laughing, dripping sweat. I drop back to my regular pace, face flushed, lungs pulling. I look back out over the city, and I think: *This is going to be fun.*

ACTIVE DATE (for 30 minutes)	CALORIES BURNED: YOU	CALORIES BURNED: HIM
Cycling (10 mph)	193	263
Dancing	145	197
Gardening	129	175
Fishing	97	131
Basketball (shooting baskets; game)	145, 258	197, 350
Bowling	97	131
Football	258	350
Golf (driving range, game)	97, 145	131, 197
Hockey (field or ice)	258	350
Horseback riding	129	175
Ice skating	226	306
Kayaking	161	219
Lacrosse	258	350
Martial arts	322	438
Rock-climbing (ascending; rappelling)	355, 258	481, 350
Rugby	322	438
Rollerblading	387	525
Scuba diving	226	306
Skiing	226	306
Sexual activity	14.5	20
Sledding	226	306
Snorkeling	161	219
Soccer (kick to kick; game)	226, 322	306, 438
Softball	193	263
Surfing	97	131
Swimming (all strokes, fast)	355	481
Tennis (doubles; singles)	161, 226	219, 306
Volleyball (game)	258	350
Walking (2 mph; 3 mph; 4 mph)	81, 106, 161	109, 144, 219

Note: Based on a 25-year-old, 5'5", 130-lb female and a 25-year-old, 5'10", 180-lb male.

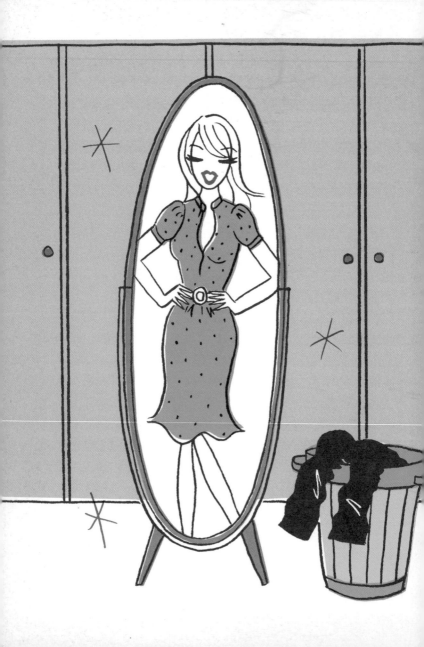

CHAPTER 10

IN THE END, IT'S UP TO YOU

Even though his mere existence tests your willpower daily, when it comes down to it, the number on the scale is your responsibility. No matter how big of a BFB you have or how many cookies, pints of ice cream, and fast-food runs he subjects you to, he's not shoving food down your throat. "What he eats drives me nuts," says Melissa, 25. "But I don't have to eat it. That's a choice I make for myself. I have a family history of heart disease and, even though I'm skinny, I have high cholesterol. I can't blame a heart attack on him because he ate chicken nuggets every day."

Although it's important to realize that his ability to eat tons of food, his willingness to dig into dessert without care, and his love of fries are dangerous to your health and your favorite jeans, it's equally necessary to look at one other very important factor: you.

Don't point an accusing finger. Realize that you are your very best ally in shedding those extra pounds or keeping them off. And that is empowering. Here are some ideas on how to check in with yourself when it comes to your own eating habits, ways to take care of yourself outside this couple entity, and what to do when you fall off the wagon.

MAKE PEACE

First of all, you must come to accept your body. Once you stop fighting it and wishing for it to turn into some airbrushed, totally unattainable magazine layout, you'll learn to listen to what your body really needs. Because if you're wanting to disown your body and totally resenting its existence, you're acting like an angry teenager who's wishing she could trade in her parents for a better set. When you're in that anger mode, you can't listen to a word they're saying, right? They're wrong, you're right, and you want nothing to do with them. It's sort of like that with your body. That doesn't mean you shouldn't set a goal to see some definition in those arms or strive for a tighter tummy; but it does mean you should stop lusting after toothpick arms or a concave, four-foot-long abdomen if you've got anything but. You can't turn into Barbie, but you can be a healthier version of yourself.

'Cause, let's face it. You're aging every day. Those arms you don't like and that butt you can't stand now are only going to sag a little bit more as you age. Sure, working out will keep you looking good for a lot longer, but it won't stop the clock. Look at your body and realize that years from now, despite all the wasted valuable minutes, hours, and days criticizing your body, you had it pretty damn good. So treat yourself with respect. And that means eating healthy and having fun. When you take care of your body, when you give it what it needs, when you don't overload it with too many calories, you naturally look and feel better.

HELLO, MY NAME IS . . .

When it comes down to it, your own food personalities—some of us have multiple issues and all are welcome here—are at the core of your unwanted boyfriend pounds. If you can pinpoint what makes you cave to his cookies or inhale half a pie with him each time you order in, you'll have a lot better chance of coming through this capable of sporting your favorite mini.

. . . And I'm a NONSTOP NOSHER

Your weakness: Oh, just about everything. Cookies, chips, candy, popcorn, an entire carton of leftover lo mein. If it's there, you'll eat it.

Recovery program: Put away, put away, put away. If you walk in and he has a bag of cookies on the counter, close the bag and stash it in the pantry. The less food lying around to tempt you, the less you'll consume.

Your mantra: Out of sight, out of mouth.

. . . .

. . . And I'm a FRUSTRATED FEEDER

Your weakness: In a word, *stress*. A fight with your (momentarily) jerk of a boyfriend, a bad day at work, or a bank account closely nose-diving toward zero are all things that can cause you to reach for ice cream—especially when your BFB is only too happy to join you.

Recovery program: Stay in tune with how you're feeling. Before putting the spoon in your mouth, pause for a moment, take a deep breath, and exhale slowly. If you still feel as anxious as a poodle on Prozac, step away from the food and crank out a few pushups, go for a run, or blare your favorite song. Anything to release some of that pent-up tension.

Your mantra: Stress sucks; tight jeans suck more!

. . . .

. . . And I'm a MARATHON MONSTER

Your weakness: You plow through the day, funneling coffee after diet soda. Come 6 P.M, you're ready to inhale whatever crap comes into view.

Recovery program: Eat small, nutrient-rich snacks throughout the day, such as an apple on the way to work, a granola bar a few hours later, and an easy-to-down lunch, like a soy smoothie or a salad with grilled chicken and low-fat dressing. You will feel a lot more even-keeled, keep that metabolism burning strong, and have much more restraint when you hit the house.

Your mantra: Day by day, snack by snack, I'll get these pounds off my back!

. . . .

. . . And I'm a SHARING SHREW

Your weakness: You live for everything to be equal and fair. You cut the sandwich down the middle, notice if his steak makes yours look puny, and if he has dessert, you have some too. You consider yourselves equals and have a tendency to make your plates look like mirror images. But unless you want a man-size belly, it's time to start giving him more when it comes to food.

Recovery program: Remind yourself that if you're half his size, your servings should be half the size of his. So serve yourself on a smaller plate and clear your plate when he starts going for seconds.

Your mantra: Less is less—on my bum!

. . . .

. . . And I'm a COMMUNAL CONSUMER

Your weakness: Eating together. Eating out, eating in—you love eating together. But besides all of that sitting and chatting, you're chewing and chewing . . . and wind up eating almost twice what you need.

Recovery program: Remember that you should be enjoying the entire event, not just the food. Notice the décor, the music, the conversation—and if you're at home, light a few candles and dim the lights to shift the focus to romance. You'll still get the best of the night—his company.

Your mantra: Eating together doesn't have to mean gaining together.

. . . .

. . . And I'm a ZONING ZOMBIE

Your weakness: Whether it's the TV, the newspaper, or total exhaustion, your hand goes to your mouth again and again, and you don't even realize it until there's nothing left on the plate.

Recovery program: Avoid your zoning area. If it's the TV, eat your main meal (starches, meat) at the table. Then, if you really enjoy your mindless munching, take your salad or veggies to the couch.

Your mantra: Don't wake up to a bigger pant size!

GUARD YOUR SLEEP

Putting sleep near the top of your to-do list may make losing those love handles a lot easier. Studies show that nonstop night owls weigh more than those who catch more shut-eye. That's because when you miss out on sleep, the body goes haywire. Ghrelin, a hormone made in the gastrointestinal tract, stimulates hunger. The less you sleep, the more ghrelin your body makes. Meanwhile, leptin—a hormone produced by the fat cells—sends signals of fullness to your brain. The less Zs you get, the less leptin you make.

Basically, when you stretch yourself to the limit and skimp on sleep, your body will get a triple whammy of bad news the next day: you'll be tired, low on leptin, and high on ghrelin—which can make you feel constantly hungry and never satisfied, no matter how much you eat. All of which can lead to overeating and making high-calorie, high-fat choices. Research shows that missing a few hours of sleep increases desire for high-carb, high-calorie food by up to 45 percent. So show that pillow some love.

HEY, YOU!

Sure, it's nice to have couple time. But between him, family, work, friends, and well, sleep, it's tough to find a few hours a week when it's just you hanging out with you. But if you want to stay happy and keep your relationship healthy, clearing out a few minutes of me time—even if it's in something as mundane as driving to the grocery store—is vital. "You can't see yourself as all-giving," says Patricia A. Farrell, PhD, author of *How to Be Your Own Therapist: A Step-by-Step Guide to Building a Competent, Confident Life*. "Helping your honey get healthy and helping yourself stay happy has to begin with you." So, think of this time as a gift you give yourself.

How much time it takes you to refill depends on your personality. If you love your bi-weekly manicures or look forward to after-work tub-soaks, good. If, however, you can't remember the last time you didn't have a human being within arm's reach or a phone attached to your ear, start to check in with yourself at least once a week. That means turning off that cell phone for an hour and curling up with a good book, blaring your favorite music and singing off-key as loudly as you please, snuggling under the covers for an oh-so-delicious Sunday afternoon nap, or heading to the mall for a few hours—by yourself. Recharge and get to know yourself better, so that you remember that alone or in a couple, there are many ways to enjoy life. You'll approach your relationship with a more secure footing, knowing who you are and why you choose to be with this person—not to mention, you'll have new things to talk about!

GIRL POWER

When you first fall head over heels, you want to spend every extra moment with your man. Unfortunately, those wonderful women—that's right, your friends—are usually moved a little bit over to the side. But those first six months or so of a new relationship pass, and suddenly you are hungry, *starving* for a no-boys-allowed, wine-filled, chocolate-eating, gossip-till-you're-passing-out girls' night. Luckily, true friends are still there—sometimes a little hurt, but, thankfully, understanding because they know they did the same thing with what's-his-name. And they are ready to catch up.

Grab a drink after work, lunch on a Saturday, or, at the very least, pick up the phone and give a girlfriend a call or send a few e-mails at least once a week. It energizes you. It reminds you that there are other people in the world who love you, who are rooting for you, who think you're fabulous (other than your mom!), and who can, well, talk about your BFB!

And don't forget, your guy needs nights out with the boys, too. "Relationships are kept alive by bringing the fun you have with others into them," says Farrell. "Think of time away as an investment in your relationship that will keep it fresh."

real-life story

Olivia, 23, loved her yoga classes. She never missed—until Mr. Wonderful showed up and she put herself on the back burner.

"I feel really good after yoga," says Olivia, who started skipping her mat sessions after she started sacrificing her evening hours—when she used to attend class—to happy coupledom. But after a few months, Olivia felt tired, unhappy, and ready to crawl out of her skin. And none of it had to do with her man! She realized she'd been neglecting her own needs for the sake of the relationship. "Yoga is one of the best feelings I've experienced; to know that you've done nothing but good for yourself for the last hour and a half, no distractions, just taking care of your mind and body." She finally decided that she needed to save time for herself in order to stay sane and happy. "It's my responsibility to make that time for myself, and I have to be strong about it!"

EAT CAKE (IF YOU REALLY WANT IT)

Life is way too short to focus on the size of your pants or what you can't be eating all the time. It's all about perspective; you never want to feel restricted or "on a diet." Don't jump to the conclusion that in order to stay thin, you have to swear off cake (or brownies, ice cream, or pasta) for life. Get to a place where you can have the cake if you really want it, but you aren't having it just because it's in front of you and cake equals happiness and birthday parties and excitement and indulgence and whatever other emotion you really want to experience at that moment. Chances are, it's not going to be found within the confines of baked goods! (No matter how good it looks, it's just flour and sugar—no fun times guaranteed!) Look for that feeling in the people instead of the cake—to the experience outside the food.

But have a piece if you really want it. Just know that there is always another slice of cake around the corner. The event is what's special, not the food attached to it. So have a bite or two, enjoy it, and realize: There is more cake to come. You don't have to finish this piece. If you really just want an apple right now, have it. You can always go get that sweet you passed up later!

I'LL GIVE YOU A SANDWICH FOR THAT COOKIE

Another thing to remember is swaps. Normally, you should look to get nutrients from carbs (see chapter 3 for a recap!), but if you're dying for a chocolate chip cookie at lunch, have a cookie at lunch! The more you resist your craving and label things taboo, the greater the chance you'll go home and eat an entire sleeve of cookies. Instead of having a sandwich *and* a cookie, eat the inside of the sandwich, leave the bread (or order a salad), and have dessert. No, you're not getting the best of nutrients, but you are balancing out the calories and carbs.

Think about compromises. If you have a carb-filled lunch, go easy at dinner—have a salad and call it a night. If you don't beat yourself up ("I'm a failure, I have no self-control"), you'll be listening to your body and realize, "Hey, I really do want these veggies! My body is actually waiting for them!"

It's a very freeing and slimming thought when you realize that nothing is "off limits," and that what you really want is balance.

NEVER GIVE UP

It *is* possible to take care of yourself and still have a fabulous time with your BFB. But nobody's perfect. You will, undoubtedly, forget this fact. One night you will find yourself eating too many fries off his plate or snacking through a bag of chips just because he left them open on the counter. When you do, pick yourself up right where you left off. Pull this book off the shelf and reread it, reminding yourself that there are thousands of other women living with BFBs and their bad habits who are going through the same thing.

Just keep at it, take care of yourself, and have fun with him—because, as crazy hard as it can be to hold onto the figure you had when you fell for him, you love him and he loves you. And *that*, as we know, isn't something to pass up seconds on.

BFB FINAL THOUGHT

Trust that you have the power to change, and don't let a boy change you.

It's another weekend, another night out. My hair is curled, pulled back in a messy updo, and as I stand in front of the mirror, dabbing on lip-gloss and spritzing my collarbone with perfume, I smile at my reflection. What a difference a few months make. My favorite jeans are now slung over a chair behind me, not because they no longer fit, but because I'm not in the mood to wear them. They've lost some of their power, now that I know I can step into them anytime I want.

I zip up a new, little black dress and bend to slide my feet into heels just as the doorbell rings. There, on the doorstep, holding a bunch of daisies and a box of chocolates, is my crazy, maddening, and all-together wonderful boyfriend. *Oh, my darling BFB.* I smile, make a mental note to toss the chocolates the second I'm home, and link my arm through his.

"You look amazing," he tells me.

A smile plays across my lips. "I know." I inhale deeply and look up at the night sky, proud of myself and excited for so much more than where we might be eating or what we'll find for dessert. The stars are out and there's no telling what the future holds.

GOOD-FOR-HIM (AND YOU!)
RECIPES

FORGET FRIED CHICKEN FINGERS

- 3 egg whites
- 3 tablespoons plain bread crumbs
- 2 tablespoons Parmesan cheese
- ½ teaspoon thyme
- ¼ teaspoon salt
- ½ teaspoon pepper
- 1 teaspoon minced onion, dried
- ½ teaspoon garlic powder
- 2 teaspoons Benefiber (optional)
- 1 pound boneless, skinless chicken tenders
- High-heat canola spray oil

Preheat oven to 350°F. Mix egg whites in small bowl and set aside. Mix all other ingredients except chicken and spray in large bowl. Dip each tender in egg whites and then roll in bread crumb mixture until well covered. Place on greased baking sheet. Spray well with high-heat canola spray. Bake 15–20 minutes or until done. Broil (about 3–5 minutes) until top becomes crispy. Serve immediately. *Serves 4.*

SO SWEET POTATO FRIES

- 1 large sweet potato
- ½ teaspoon salt
- 1 teaspoon cinnamon
- 2 teaspoons sugar or stevia
- High-heat canola cooking spray

Preheat oven to 425°F. Wash sweet potato with soap and water; rinse thoroughly. Mix salt, cinnamon, and sugar in a small bowl, and set aside. Cut sweet potato in half lengthwise, and then cut it into fry-length wedges. Place wedges in large bowl. Spray generously with high-heat canola cooking spray, tossing until wedges are evenly coated. Toss again with spice mixture, making sure all wedges are coated with spices. Place wedges on greased baking sheet, spreading them out evenly. Spray wedges again with canola spray. Bake in oven 20–25 minutes or until soft. Serve immediately. *Serves 2.*

BETTER-FOR-YOU BURGERS

- ½ cup frozen (or fresh) onions, chopped
- ½ cup frozen (or fresh) peppers, chopped
- 1 pound extra-lean ground beef
- ½ cup rolled oats
- ½ cup low-sodium V8
- 1 teaspoon garlic powder
- Salt and pepper, to taste

Microwave frozen peppers and onions in small bowl, about 1 minute. Drain. Mix together all ingredients in large bowl. Mash with a fork, making sure oats and vegetables are thoroughly combined. Shape into firm patties. Grill until done to taste. *Serves 4–6.*

GIMME GINGER BROCCOLI*

- 1 tablespoon olive oil
- ¼ cup frozen (or fresh) onions, diced
- One 16-ounce bag frozen broccoli
- Low-sodium soy sauce, to taste
- ½ teaspoon of ginger
- ½ teaspoon of garlic

Drizzle oil in large nonstick skillet. Place skillet on medium-high heat. Once hot, add onions. Allow onions to brown, about 2 minutes. Add broccoli, stirring to prevent sticking. Drizzle with soy sauce. Add ginger and garlic. Stir until combined, adding a little water if broccoli appears to be sticking. Cover and allow to cook, stirring occasionally, until broccoli is done, about 7 to 10 minutes. *Serves 4.*

*This recipe can also be made with chicken cooked with olive oil, onions, and spices for 5 minutes. Then add broccoli and cook for 2–3 minutes more.

BANGIN' BUFFALO CHICKEN TENDERS

- 1 lb. boneless skinless chicken tenders
- 1 bottle (12 oz) Louisiana hot sauce
- 1 teaspoon paprika
- 1 teaspoon ground hot peppers

Preheat oven to 350°F. Rinse chicken and cut off any last bits of fat. Cut into thin, one-inch strips. Lay in shallow glass dish. Pour hot sauce over chicken until covered. Add paprika and hot peppers and move chicken around until spices are mixed. Place in oven for about 15–20 minutes or until chicken is thoroughly cooked. Serve with celery sticks and fat-free ranch dressing or low-fat bleu cheese dressing. *Serves 4–6.*

POWER PANCAKES

....

- ½ cup 100% white whole-wheat flour
- 1 cup fat-free Greek yogurt
- 4 egg whites
- 1 tablespoon canola oil
- ½ cup applesauce or mashed bananas
- 1 tablespoon baking powder
- 1 tablespoon vanilla
- 1 teaspoon cinnamon
- 2 teaspoons Benefiber (optional)
- Any other chopped or pureed fruit you'd like: blueberries, bananas, chunks of thinly sliced apple, raspberries, etc.
- Agave nectar (instead of syrup)

Mix all the ingredients (except the agave nectar) in a large mixing bowl. Stir until thoroughly combined, about 1 minute. Spray skillet with nonstick spray and heat over medium-high on stove. Wait until pan is hot enough that water bubbles when flicked onto surface. Spoon one large tablespoon (the batter spreads out quite a bit) onto skillet for each pancake. Allow to cook until pancake is bubbling in the center. Flip and cook until done; Cook slower and longer than regular pancakes to ensure middle is thoroughly cooked. Heat agave nectar in microwave about 30 seconds, then drizzle over the pancakes. Yum! *Serves 4–6.*

BETTER-THAN-COOKIES
BAKED OATMEAL

- 2 cups skim milk
- ½ cup canola oil
- ½ cup all natural apple butter spread or applesauce (no sugar added)
- 1 large egg
- 4 large egg whites
- ½ cup agave nectar
- ¼ cup brown sugar
- 2 tablespoons cinnamon
- 1 tablespoon vanilla
- 4 teaspoons baking powder
- Stevia, to taste
- Cinnamon, to taste
- 6 cups rolled oats
- Handful of raisins or chopped apples (optional)

Preheat oven to 350°F. Combine all ingredients except oats in a large mixing bowl. Stir well, making sure to remove nearly all lumps. Add oats. Pour into 13x9-inch greased baking pan. Sprinkle with stevia and cinnamon. Bake 25 minutes or until a toothpick inserted in the center comes out clean. Eat within two days, or cut into squares, wrap in wax paper, place in freezer bags, and freeze. To defrost, pop them into the microwave for about 1 minute for a wonderful, warm snack.
Serves 12–16.

BEST BOOTY BERRY SMOOTHIE

- ½ cup cottage cheese
- ½ cup frozen blueberries
- ½ cup frozen strawberries
- 1 teaspoon vanilla
- ½ cup water
- 1 tablespoon vanilla whey protein
(sweetened with stevia)
- Crushed ice to taste (depending on
how thick you want it)

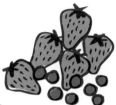

Place cottage cheese, berries, vanilla,
and a dash of water in a blender. Blend well.
(You may need to add more water to get things moving.)
Add whey protein powder. Blend until smooth. If not
thick or cold enough, add crushed ice. Continue adding
ice or water until the mixture reaches the desired consistency. Some people like smoothies thin enough to sip;
others love them just as thick and creamy as ice cream.
One serving.

TABLE OF
EQUIVALENCIES

VOLUME

UNITED STATES	METRIC
⅛ teaspoon	1.25 ml
¼ teaspoon	2.5 ml
1 teaspoon	5 ml
1 tablespoon (3 teaspoons)	15 ml
1 fl oz (2 tablespoons)	30 ml
¼ cup	60 ml
⅓ cup	80 ml
½ cup	120 ml
1 cup	240 ml
1 pint (2 cups)	480 ml
1 quart (2 pints)	960 ml
1 gallon (4 quarts)	3.84 liters

WEIGHT

UNITED STATES	METRIC
1 oz	28 g
4 oz (¼ lb)	113 g
8 oz (½ lb)	227 g
12 oz (¾ lb)	340 g
16 oz (1 lb)	454 g
2.2 lb	1 kg

OVEN TEMPERATURES

DEGREES FAHRENHEIT	DEGREES CENTIGRADE	BRITISH GAS MARKS
200	93	—
250	120	½
275	140	1
300	150	2
325	165	3
350	175	4
375	190	5
400	200	6
450	230	8
500	260	10

LENGTH

INCHES	CENTIMETERS
¼	0.65
½	1.25
1	2.50
2	5.00
3	7.50
4	10.0
5	12.5
6	15.0
7	17.5
8	20.5
9	23.0
10	25.5
12	30.5
15	38.0

SELECTED SOURCES

BOOKS AND ARTICLES

Anders, Mark. "ACE-Sponsored Research Study: Human Joysticks." *Fitness Matters* 13, no. 5 (2007): 7–9.

Burke, Edmund. *Precision Heart Rate Training*. Champaign, IL: Human Kinetics Publishers, 1998.

Carper, Jean. "Garlic's Breath of Health." *USA Weekend Magazine*, April 2, 1995.

Christakis, Nicholas A., et al. "The Spread of Obesity in a Large Social Network Over 32 Years." *The New England Journal of Medicine* 357, no. 4 (2007): 370–379.

Finkelstein E. A., L. A. Linnan, D. F. Tate, and B. E. Birken. "A Pilot Study Testing the Effect of Different Levels of Financial Incentives on Weight Loss Among Overweight Employees." *Journal of Occupational and Environmental Medicine* 49, no. 9: (2007): 981–989.

Johnston C. S., C. M. Kim, and A. J. Buller. "Vinegar Improves Insulin Sensitivity to a High-Carbohydrate Meal in Subjects with Insulin Resistance or Type 2 Diabetes." *Diabetes Care* 27 (2004): 281–282.

Lake, Amelia. "Could Your Partner Be Bad for Your Health?" *Complete Nutrition* (2006): 8–11.

Levitsky, David A. and Trisha Youn. "The More Food Young Adults are served, the More they Overeat." *Journal of Nutrition* 134 (2004): 2546–2549.

Platkin, Charles Stuart. "Flavorful Seasonings That Spice Up Health Benefits." The *Seattle Times*, July 27, 2005.

Raynor, Douglas A. *et al*. "Television Viewing and Long-Term Weight Maintenance: Results from the National Weight Control Registry." *Obesity* 14, no. 10 (2006): 1816–1824.

Squires, Sally. "Olive Oil: The Slippery Details." The *Washington Post*, November 9, 2004.

WEB SITES

See individual company web sites for more nutrition information on their products.

American Heart Association. "Saturated Fats." September 2007, http://www.americanheart.org/presenter.jhtml?identifier=3045790.

Associated Press. "Thin People May Be Fat on the Inside, Doctors Warn." May 11,

2007, http://www.cbc.ca/health/story/2007/05/11/fat-internal.html.

Bouchez, Colette. "Exercise Your Body—and Your Skin." *WebMD*, May 6, 2005, http://www.webmd.com/skin-beauty/guide/exercise-your-body-your-skin.

———. "The Dream Diet: Losing Weight While You Sleep." *WebMD*, 1 Jan. 2007, http://www.webmd.com/sleep-disorders/guide/lose-weight-while-sleeping

———. "Yoga for Weight Loss?" *MedicineNet*, July 21, 2006, http://www.medicinenet.com/script/main/art.asp?articlekey=63034.

"Calorie King Food & Exercise Diary," *CalorieKing.com*, http://www.calorieking.com/tools/exercise_calories.php.

Center for Disease Control and Prevention. "About BMI for Adults." May 22, 2007. http://www.cdc.gov/nccdphp/dnpa/bmi/adult_BMI/about_adult_BMI.htm.

———. "Chapter 2 Conclusions." *Physical Activity and Health: A Report of the Surgeon General*. May 2008, http://www.cdc.gov/nccdphp/sgr/chapcon.htm.

Center for Food and Safety and Applied Nutrition. "A Food Labeling Guide—Appendix A: Definitions of Nutrient Content Claims," April 2008. http://www.cfsan.fda.gov/~dms//21g-xa.html.

Collins, Karen. "Olive Oil Brings More than Flavor to Your Diet." *MSNBC*, April 4, 2006, http://www.msnbc.msn.com/id/11758647.

Cox, Amy. "Exercise: Key to Good Sex, Good Sleep." CNN, May 28, 2007, http://edition.cnn.com/2006/HEALTH/diet.fitness/06/20/hb.exercise.benefits/index.html.

Crary, David. "Men Who Do Housework May Get More Sex, " *Live Science*, March 6, 2008, http://www.livescience.com/health/080306-ap-men-housework.html.

Cromie, William J. "Exercise Cuts Risk of Sudden Cardiac Death." *Harvard Gazette*, March 23, 2006, http://www.news.harvard.edu/gazette/2006/03.23/05-suddendeath.html.

DeNoon, Daniel. "Dark Chocolate Is Healthy Chocolate." *WebMD*, August 27, 2003, http://www.webmd.com/diet/news/20030827/dark-chocolate-is-healthy-chocolate.

———. "Drink More Diet Soda, Gain More Weight?" *WebMD*, June 13, 2005, http://www.webmd.com/diet/news/20050613/drink-more-diet-soda-gain-more-weight.

"Harris Benedict Equation." *BMI Calculator*, http://www.bmi-calculator.net/bmr-calculator/harris-benedict-equation.

"How many calories do you burn during?" *FITDAY*, http://www.fitday.com/webfit/exerciseinfopage.html.

Jordan, Jaime. "The Amazing No-Gym Workout!" *Time Out New York*, January 10, 2008, http://www.timeout.com/newyork/articles/features/25527/the-amazing-no-gym-workout.

Kozolchyk, Abbie. "Best Sugar Substitutes." *Body + Soul*, April 2008. http://www.marthastewart.com/article/healthy-sugar-substitutes.

Lake, Amelia. "Cohabiting is Bad for Women's Health—But Not Men's." *Complete Nutrition*, April 5, 2006, http://www.ncl.ac.uk/press.office/press.release/content.phtml?ref=1144224014.

Lempert, Phil. "Stevia is the New Splenda." *Supermarket Guru on iVillage*. March 26, 2008, http:/supermarketguru.ivillage.com/food/archives/2008/03/stevia-is-the-new-splenda.html.

Margolin, Evan. "Salsa Dancing Burns Calories." *Ezine* Articles, http://ezinearticles.com/?Salsa-Dancing-Burns-Calories&id=232313.

Nelson, Miriam. "Does When You Work Out Determine How Many Calories You Burn? *CNN*, July 14, 1999, http://www.cnn.com/HEALTH/diet.fitness/9907/14/workout.times/index.html.

Nissl, Jan. "Men's Health: Testosterone." *WebMD*, June, 13, 2006, http://men.webmd.com/testosterone-15738.

Pick, Marcelle. "Sugar Substitutes and the Potential Danger of Splenda." *Women to Women*. January 15, 2008, http://www.womentowomen.com/nutritionandweightloss/splenda.aspx

Pizzorno, Joseph. "Integrative Medicine and Wellness: Ah, Roughage." *WebMD*, October 16, 2007, http://blogs.webmd.com/integrative-medicine-wellness/2007/10/ah-roughage.html.

"Protein 101: How much do you need?" *TODAY*, August 29, 2006, http://www.msnbc.msn.com/id/14563169.

"Raise a Pint: Scientists Say Beer Has Essential Cancer-Fighting Agents" *Fox News*, January 14, 2008, http://www.foxnews.com/story/0,2933,322571,00.html.

Simmons, Michele. "The Health Benefits of Garlic." *iVillage*, March 15, 2008, http://www.ivillage.co.uk/health/comp/herb/articles/0,181042_183722,00.html.

Villareal, D. T. and J. O. Holloszy. "Stomach Fat and Insulin Resistance." *American Diabetes Association*, 2004, http://www.diabetes.org/diabetes-research/summaries/villareal-stomach.jsp.

Warner, Jennifer. "Exercise Fights Fatigue, Boosts Energy." *WebMD*, November 3, 2006, http://www.webmd.com/diet/news/20061103/exercise-fights-fatigue-boosts-energy.

Zelman, Kathleen. "How Accurate Is Body Mass Index, or BMI?" *WebMD*, 2007, http://www.webmd.com/diet/features/how-accurate-body-mass-index-bmi.

USDA. "Chapter 7: Carbohydrates." *USDA Dietary Guidelines for Americans 2005*, http://www.health.gov/dietaryguidelines/dga2005/document/html/chapter7.htm.

INDEX

ACKNOWLEDGMENTS

Thank you to all the wonderful people who made this book possible:

Sarah O'Brien, my editor, who believed in *BFB* from the very first email, and who convinced the rest of the amazingly talented Quirk team that we had to write it.

Molly Lyons, my agent: I am so lucky to have you on my team.

The experts who shared their time and knowledge: Amelia Lake, Kathleen Zelman, Brooke Hayward, Patricia A. Farrell, Anne Volk, and Connie Holt, for looking over the book with a dietitian's eye.

Elena Chin and Marielle Messing for fact-checking the book.

Everyone at *Philadelphia* magazine, especially Emily Gagne, Jane Morley, Carrie Denny, and Timothy Haas.

My family: Mom, Julie, Joe, Joy, and Jessica; my second family: MaryAnn, Jon, Josh, and Steve Gerben; Grandpa and all the Genevies. You are my world and I love you all.

Emily Martin, Jill Waldbieser, Jammie Williams, Erin Garwood, Laura McIntosh, Kelly and Erin Zimmerman, Randi Olley, Courtney Knauss, Susan, Steven, and Carly, Dhruv Wadhwa, Gary and Karol Myers, Elke and Bud Gerben, the Greenfield family, the 6 A.M. coffee Spin club, and anyone else my overworked brain may have missed: Your support means more than you will ever know.

The hysterical and inspiring women who shared stories of life with their BFB: Please stay in touch! bigfatboyfriend@yahoo.com

And, of course, my BFB: Thank you for actually believing this book was a good idea (even if it meant enduring countless jokes about your "weight problem"—you deserve an award!). I love you, french fries and all.